John P. Lenhart M.D.

HAPPY LIFE

HEALTHY
AGING

John P. Lenhart M.D.

Front Cover Photo – Cape Spear Newfoundland

Photographer – John P. Lenhart MD

Editors – May Collins and Lauren Lenhart

I would like to thank my editors for helping make this book easier to read. Through their effort a more polished manuscript was made possible.

HAPPY LIFE
HEALTHY
AGING

JOHN P LENHART MD

John P. Lenhart M.D.

ISBN #:   Softcover   978-1-930822-33-7

This book was printed in the United States of America.

To order additional copies of this book, contact:
www.happylifehealthyaging.com
www.amazon.com
Medfo Publishing
St Petersburg, Florida

CONTENTS

John P. Lenhart M.D.

DISCLAIMER

This book is not intended to act as a substitute for advice from your personal physician. The information presented in this book is for educational purposes only and not intended to diagnose or treat disease, nor to render medical advice. Before starting any longevity program, please consult your personal physician to determine the appropriateness of that program based upon your personal medical history.

The information in this book was derived from personal experiences of the author, original research, other books on similar subjects, basic research papers, researching individuals, and from anti-aging seminars and lectures at the American College for Advancement in Medicine.

Introduction

A number of years ago, a book titled *Passages* was written. It described the stages of life we go through as we pass through this beautiful earth of ours. Our time is only a fraction of a blink in the grand scheme of things. The Milky Way galaxy in which we live has billions of stars just like our sun, and the universe is filled with billions of galaxies just like our own. When peering into the infinite space of our universe, one begins to grasp how minuscule our existence truly is.

Our existence is finite. How we can maximize our potential to get the full benefit of this earth is what this book is about. I want you to have a happy life with healthy aging. No one can guarantee anything in this life, but by using existing knowledge we can try to increase our chances to achieve that healthy aging goal. This is not a trial run, you have to think things through and plan what you want to do and implement that plan in the final third of your life.

After years of education and research, I have accumulated the knowledge and understanding of what it truly means to live to the fullest. Through *Happy Life Healthy Aging*, I hope to share this information with others, maximizing your chances of healthy aging and a happy life. Few things in this life happen by chance. You had to put in a lot of effort to get to the stage in life you are in now. In retirement the same rules apply. Having lived in Florida for a long time, I have seen many passages. The health and lifestyle choices people made in those passages made a huge difference in their ability to enjoy the fruits of their labor.

My mission in life now, as a semi-retired doctor, is to keep all of you as healthy and as happy as possible. The principles laid down in this book, I believe, are vital in your quest for that "Happy Life in Healthy Aging"

May you be happy, healthy, wise, prosperous, successful and in love with your life on this earth. Best wishes on your journey.

Dr. John P. Lenhart

John P. Lenhart M.D.

FOREWORD

There's a revolution going on, one that is slowly creeping into the psyche of the American experience; one that is not about money, political ideals, social justice or power.

This is an internal revolution driven by a biological clock. We're not willing to settle for the ticking away of life. We're not content to sit by while our bodies shrivel, our minds forget, and our sexual potency is lost.

WE WANT TO STAY YOUNG FOREVER!

This revolution is in the spirit of Life. It is the Life Force that makes us what we are, and our reactions that give our inner selves feelings of action, exuberance, and ecstasy.

We Baby Boomers have seen our grandparents rock away their lives in rocking chairs, our parents vegetate before the T.V. We've seen them turn old, long before their time. We've seen them become incapacitated, relegated to nursing homes, and suffer massive infections due to bed sores, heart disease, diabetes, and other chronic ailments that rob them of the essence of Life.

We Baby Boomers say, NO! There must be a better way to live when we're old.

And there is. *Happy Life Healthy Aging* explores the options available that are known to increase life, vitality, memory, and mobility, and avoid many of the pitfalls associated with aging. There has been an explosion of knowledge and interest in anti-aging. This book encapsulates this knowledge in simple terms easily understood by the layperson. You can read this book in depth or you can skim it over to get the most essential ideas.

At whatever level you read *Happy Life Healthy Aging*, you will gain from it and become a healthier individual, avoiding many of the pitfalls that devoured our parents and grandparents as they aged.

We pamper our pets, we pamper our cars, we pamper our boats but why have we abused our bodies? In the first half of our lives our bodies take care of us, but in the second half of our lives we have to take care of our bodies.

If we take care of our bodies and mind, they will give us good service and pleasure in life. You can do it at any stage of your life; the body is very resilient and can repair itself as outlined in this book. We are very fortunate to have such a wonderful machine working for us, nursing us along through all the abuses we throw at it, but there is a limit to how much abuse the body can stand.

The *Happy Life Healthy Aging* book gives you a logical, easy to understand system of changes you can make that will reverse the aging process as much as possible. When you take control of your biological clock, you realize that healthy aging is a reality and that you can have a healthy, happy, active last half of your life without physical or mental impediments.

If you implement just one of the *Healthy Aging* secrets you will have great anti-aging benefits, but when you stack them together watch out! Your energy level will go through the roof and you will feel forty again.

So become a revolutionary, take control, take charge of your life, and reverse your aging process.

Have fun in life and enjoy the benefits of a *Happy Life and Healthy Aging*.

John P. Lenhart M.D.

CHAPTER 1

The Secrets of a Happy Life and Healthy Aging

You're starting to feel a little older, aren't you? You're thinking more about aging now, especially when you look in the mirror. You compare yourself to friends your own age, and secretly see how they measure up to you.

Why do you suppose you feel that way? Is there something inside you that says, "There must be something I can do about it?" Is that what made you want to read this book? Or, did a friend tell you that following its suggestions made profound changes in his life?

For whatever reason, the best thing you've ever done to help delay the aging process was to pick up and start reading this book.

You're obviously not the average individual who allows time and the natural environment determine your fate, growing old without a fight. Not you. You want to stay active. You want to stay mentally alert. You want to stay strong and vigorous. And, you want to remain interested in exploring the world and all of its possibilities well into your old age without physical restrictions.

You want to *LIVE* and not let the world pass you by as you bide your time until you hit the grave.

One good thing about healthy aging is that **it is never too late to start.** You can begin a longevity program from any age, beginning in your 30s right through to your 90s.

Back in the late 1970s, I started practicing preventative medicine. After I received my first doctoral degree, and additionally training in acupuncture and nutrition, I began observing the changes people made in their lives that affected them in their later years. Through that process of observation, reading, attending numerous seminars, as well as seeing thousands of patients, I have been able to deduce certain qualities that are essential in preserving a healthy, vigorous life well into old age.

In spending a considerable amount of time studying many phases of medicine, traditional as well as non-traditional, I have observed key components that make a significant difference in how patients age.

Offering alternative/complementary options for patients' conditions that reduced, and many times eliminated, the need for drugs and invasive surgery over the years, I've observed that many of these conditions are totally preventable, especially chronic degenerative diseases that plague society today.

I've also noticed that starting at almost any age, it is possible to reverse the downhill spiral of aging and live a vigorous, healthy lifestyle well into the 80's and 90's.

Theoretically, it is possible to maintain an active, healthy lifestyle past 100 or even 120 years of age. But, if I said you could be healthy at 120 or 150, you wouldn't believe me, would you? So, let's not get farfetched. Let's make things easily understandable and attainable. We want to have a healthy and vigorous lifestyle well into our 80s and 90s.

Some things in this book you will believe and others you will doubt, which is normal in human nature. Things you doubt, you need to research on the internet yourself. Our references will be posted on our web site happylifehealthyaging.com. Be careful, not all information posted on the internet is always true. Go to the NIH (National Institute of Health) or NCCIH (The National Center for Complementary and Integrative Health) web sites. Research-recognized peer-reviewed journals such as *JAMA Journal of the American Medical Association, Scientific American, Nutrition, Annals of Internal Medicine, Lancet, NEJM New England Journal of Medicine*, and the Cochrane Collaboration. Unless an article has been peer-reviewed and gone under intense scrutiny by fellow scientists, it can be very misleading and not accurate. Even peer-reviewed articles are sometimes later retracted if the data cannot be replicated by someone else.

So, what are the secrets of a happy life and healthy aging? Based upon my clinical experience, observing patients throughout their lifetimes, extensive literature research, experience teaching other physicians about anti-aging, and my broad training in medicine, integrative medicine, alternative medicine, chiropractic, as well as acupuncture and homeopathy, I have been able to derive key components essential for a healthy longevity program. Each of these components will be described in individual chapters, and further excerpts are available in the reference section of the book. You can also use Google Scholar.

Here are the healthy aging secrets:

1. **Clean Out/Detoxify Your Body** – Over the years, the body accumulates thousands of toxins that it can only partially eliminate or not eliminate at all. These toxins leave residue that slowly accumulate in the body, sludging up our system and preventing us from metabolizing and working properly. The

gradual, toxic, biological and chemical sludge that accumulates in our systems slowly bogs down those chemical and electrical processes that allow our bodies to function normally. This interference eventually leads to the chronic diseases prevalent in today's society, such as cardiovascular disease, circulatory problems, Alzheimer's disease, cancer, diabetes, arthritis, and numerous other chronic conditions.

2. **Happy things to do in Healthy Aging** – In order to be happy, we have to do activities that bring us joy. Happy things increase our endorphins, the little pleasure chemicals in our brain. To truly live means to enjoy life to its fullest and fulfill our passions. This chapter discusses possible activities to pursue that we had no time for in our working years, and exposes you to activities you may never have thought of.

3. **Caloric Restriction** – Since 1991, the incidence of obesity in the United States has tripled. BIG FAT is winning, making a lot of corporations very wealthy. The price on our health that BIG FAT exacts is catastrophic. There are scores of diseases associated with obesity and overweight conditions. These diseases are gradual in onset, rob us of our youthfulness, and gradually induce inactivity, chronic diseases, immobility, and death. There are numerous, well-documented, studies that show that caloric restriction is one of the healthiest lifestyles for promoting longevity, mobility, and mental acuteness. As a nation, we're eating ourselves to death. If this process doesn't stop, we'll be unable to afford to pay for the chronic conditions we will endure in our lifetime and will suffer in misery in our old age.

The good news is that this obesity cycle can be reversed. You can regain good health while at the same time improving your life quality and longevity.

4. **Physical Activity and Longevity** – Through my experience as a preventative-minded physician, I've seen numerous patients at death's door, pale, weak, and frail, who then, through physical activity and exercise, totally reverse that state. They become vigorous, active, clear-thinking senior citizens with good muscle tone, agility, and stamina. Numerous studies throughout the world have shown that physical activity can significantly reduce all disease processes, including cancer, and at the same time increase our life span as well as greatly enhance our quality of life.

5. **Vitamins, Minerals, Herbs, and Anti-Oxidants**
(This might be the hardest chapter to read in this book so you may want to read it in snippets.)

In the 1970's when I was practicing preventative medicine (known as holistic medicine at that time), other doctors scoffed at the money patients were "wasting" on vitamins and minerals. I knew the data was out there. I read basic research from the 1930s and 40s. However, the majority of the medical community was not aware of it and stated that you got all the vitamins and minerals you needed from the food you ate. Taking anything else in addition was a waste of money. How times have changed. Nowadays you see vitamins and minerals constantly advertised on television. Now there's an ongoing consensus that our food is devoid of necessary vitamins and minerals due to the depletion of nutrients in our soil. Over twenty years, after I first recommended vitamins and minerals, the mainstream medical community slowly has started to change its opinion on the need for supplementation because the public demanded it. There are well designed studies available now. The general public has found that by supplementing daily food intake with necessary vitamins and minerals, they may feel better and may prevent some of the ailments of modern society by giving their bodies optimized nutrition. Antioxidants have recently been found to prevent free radical damage. Thirty years ago no one had heard of free radicals that slowly destroy our cells. The more we learn about the body, the more we realize that we need specific vitamins, minerals and essential fatty acids for optimization of our health.

6. **Hormone Replacements** – Human growth hormone (HGH) and other naturally occurring hormones have only recently been used on an off-label basis to enhance the appearance of youth and vitality. The original studies done in the early 1990's by Dr. Dennis Rudman documented the antiaging effects of growth hormone on our muscles, fat tissue, and overall appearance and energy and stamina. Natural hormone replacements for postmenopausal females, and some for males, trickled into mainstream medicine and the media. **However, newer studies advise caution. The risks may outweigh the results.** This chapter and our web site: happylifehealthyaging.com may help you to decide what direction to take.

7. **Fruits, Vegetables, and Dietary Choices** – The old saying, "Garbage in, garbage out," couldn't be more true in our biological systems. What we take in is what we get out of it. In general, when we consume foods poor in nutrients the building blocks that build our body are going to be very, very poor. Poor building blocks in our cells, bones, nerve tissues, and muscles make them very susceptible to disease processes. This decreased immunity increases our susceptibility to various diseases, including cancers. What held true for the three little pigs and the big bad wolf in the book "Little Red Riding Hood" holds true for our bodies. The house the pig built out of brick withstood the huffing and puffing of the big bad wolf. That pig survived. However, the houses built of weak materials were blown over and the wolf ate those pigs. Just think about it: Doesn't cancer eat us up just like the wolf ate the pigs in the weak houses? What kind of house do you want to have? The stronger your immune system, the more resistance you have to chronic diseases.

8. The Healthy Mind – Active, Happy and Stress Free.

Our psychological input is just as important to our health as our physical input. "Garbage in, garbage out," is just as meaningful in our emotions and our psychological well-being as it is in the diet that we eat. A number of years ago, Dr. Hans Selye, a prominent Canadian physician, was able to replicate many of the chronic degenerative conditions and diseases that plague us today by stressing animals to the point that their immune systems started breaking down. The result? The animals developed numerous physical ailments. The only variation was the stress placed upon the animals. We know from experience that our mental state exerts a large influence on our physical well-being.

Visualization and laughter therapy have even been used for cancer treatment with success. Reduced stress, happy thoughts, happy relationships, love, and plenty of time for play are essential for the prolongation of life in healthy human beings. I have had friends who were senior executives in corporations with their own private jets tell me, "I got out of this rat race. If I had stayed in, I would be dead like the rest of my friends." They are now leading happy retired lives in Florida, playing as much as possible and enjoying life. Happy thoughts, and things we do while being socially engaged, are essential for longevity.

In the following chapters, I will go over the key components to a happy life and healthy aging. I will give you particulars as to the amount, duration, time, and dosage ranges, including specific dietary recommendations, exercise regimens, and many other useful hints that may help prolong your life and increase its quality.

Chapter 2

Happy Things to do in Healthy Aging

This chapter did not exist in the *Seven Secrets of Anti-Aging* book. When talking to retirees, I noticed that some did not have hobbies or interests outside of their work. Many professionals were so engrossed in their work that they had little time to develop other interests. By reading this chapter, you may get some ideas of things to try that will bring you pleasure in retirement and a happier life.

We humans are creatures of emotion. We make major decisions based on emotion. Our religious beliefs, the partner we marry, our political affiliation and our career and leisure time activities all have an emotional component. When we retire we want to have as many positive emotions as possible and reduce or eliminate the negative ones. By focusing on "living happily", we accentuate the positives and try to eliminate the negatives in our lives.

What does "to live" mean? For me it means passion. That spark and life that stimulates us to go on and achieve new goals, new pleasures and new joys. It means to spark new desires yet to be fulfilled. It is an intense burning to achieve something or do something that you find infinitely rewarding. And please note, there's a big difference between "existing" and "living".

To "live" means reaching beyond the ordinary, beyond just mere existence. It means exploring those passions that before retirement you never had the time to do because ordinary life got in the way. Now is the time to let go, explore and enjoy those things you dreamed of doing. This is the final quarter of your life game, have fun and enjoy these "Happy things to do in Healthy Aging":

1. **The Morning Walk** – Taking a walk the first thing in the morning is a good thing to do. It gets you moving, smell the fresh air, watch the sunrise, burn calories and makes you feel good about yourself.

2. **The Night Walk**– Everyone loves a sunset. Why not combine watching a sunset with a half hour walk before and after the sun actually sets when the colors become spectacular..

3. **Going to the Gym** –Friends of mine go to the Y several times per week and love the classes. In North America we have huge gym complexes with everything imaginable in them. In my building there are always people working out on the treadmill, weight machines or free weights. They enjoy staying in shape, and keeping their muscles toned.

4. **Bike Rides** – We have many bicycling clubs in St Petersburg, Florida. I belong to a rollerblade and biking group and we have different rides three times per week. We meet up at various locations and do 11-15 mile rides. I also ride my road bike with serious gearheads. You do not have to go fast, just get out and enjoy bike riding at whatever level you feel comfortable. It helps if your city has numerous biking trails as they have in Sopot, Poland, Berlin, Germany or Belgium.

5. **Bible/Spiritual Study Groups** – Numerous people get involved in bible/spiritual study. They want to understand their religion better. The inner peace that people find from religious studies makes them happy. Spirituality and having a connection with God is very important to many.

6. **Sailing** – Being anywhere by the water makes many people happy. Many of my friends love to go sailing on beautiful sunny, windy days just like I do. Albert Einstein was a big fan of sailing, that is where he did his most inspirational thinking. Walter Cronkite was also an avid sailor and so is Morgan

Freeman. Yacht racing, or learning to crew by joining a sailing club, can be challenging and a lot of fun as well.

7. **Bridge Clubs** – In Florida there are many Bridge card clubs at the Masters level. People find Bridge to be an enjoyable strategic card game that can be socially engaging as well. Many other card games are also popular. Mah Jongg is also gaining in popularity.

8. **Kayaking** – Kayaking is something that I like to do on a regular basis. It is one of the cheapest forms of boating that you can do. Kayaks are portable and can be enjoyed on lakes, rivers and oceans. Join a kayaking club and have fun exploring.

9. **Tennis / Pickleball** – Tennis is very popular in warm climates. It is an aerobic and social activity requiring strategy and skill. Make sure that you are playing on soft courts not concrete. Your knees will last much longer if you play on har-tru green clay courts. In St Petersburg, Florida, we have pick-up round-robin tennis on Monday, Wednesday, and Friday mornings where you switch doubles partners every third game. It's a no-brainer, get out of bed, be there by 8:30 and there is a group of tennis players waiting to play. Pickleball is a transition from tennis into a smaller court and played a lot in retirement communities, as is Ping Pong.

10. **Baseball League** – All cities have baseball leagues. Find a senior league and start playing. Senior soccer is also an option.

11. **Golfing Group** – Retirement and golfing go hand in hand. You will find hundreds of communities designed around golf courses in many towns. Some will also have aerobics classes, a gym, guest lectures and excellent dining facilities.

12. **Trail Hiking** – My niece in Europe loves to go hiking in the mountains. She belongs to a hiking group and every weekend there is a trip planned somewhere for all-day hikes. Hiking is a great way to exercise and experience nature as you watch the flowers bloom or animals frolic in the meadows and woods.

13. **Dancing** – My book "**Dance to Live**" points out the health benefits of dancing. In my opinion dancing is one of the best activities for aerobic exercise, balance, coordination, mental enhancement, stress reduction and social engagement all

wrapped up into one fun-filled activity. In my area there are large, weekly east coast swing dances with lessons, Argentine tango, Carolina shag, salsa, square and contra dances, as well as multiple ballroom dances at various studios. I know a couple in their late 70s who dance 5 nights a week. He picks her up and twirls her around as if they were 20 again. I also dance with a lovely 87 year old lady who is convinced that dancing keeps her young, and I agree.

14. **Date Nights** – Just as dating was important when you were raising children, dating is important in retirement. It keeps you engaged with your partner while having fun doing those activities you both enjoy together. Your date could be the traditional dinner and a movie, or an evening performance at the theatre or symphony. Anyplace where the two of you have time to connect and enjoy each other's company is ideal.

15. **Girls' Night Out** – Girls need their night out, just to be girls again and have fun without worrying about what the guys think.

16. **Guys' Night Out** – Guys love to get together in their man-caves and solve the world's problems. They also love to get together to talk about their hobbies and sport teams.

17. **Fishing** – I've known many fishermen that get up at 4AM to catch that incoming tide or go out on their flatboats. Fly fishing can become a passion for some people and they will travel half way around the world to do it. Offshore fishing is very popular in Florida, as is lake fishing.

18. **Shooting and Archery** – From clay pigeon shooting to target practice, shooting has been a hobby and sport for thousands of years. Archery, the original form of shooting, is also still popular.

19. **Jewelry Making** – A retired psychiatrist I knew had an entire room dedicated to bead jewelry making. She loved to make glass and colored stone necklaces and bracelets. She found it to be relaxing as well as creative.

20. **Painting, Pottery and Ceramics** – Many people have always wanted to paint but never had the time to do it. Now is the time to take that art class and learn what you can do. Making

stained glass windows is another hobby that retirees are taking up along with throwing clay pots and decorative ceramic glazing.

21. **Knitting and Sewing** – A friend of mine developed a second career after retiring, designing specialty yarns and writing knitting books that became very successful. Look for a sewing meet-up group and explore designing your own clothes.

22. **Racquet Ball** – Just like tennis, racquet ball is a competitive aerobic sport that gives you fast paced work outs and an opportunity to socialize. **Badminton** can also be very competitive.

23. **Book Clubs** – Reading is very popular for many people. In St Petersburg, Florida, there is a "Festival of Reading" that brings authors from everywhere to talk about their books and what inspired them. Book clubs get together to select a book of the month to read and discuss that book at their next meeting. The meetings are generally at someone's home and are quite enjoyable.

24. **Travel Clubs** – In retirement, many people love to travel. They want to visit places that they have read about to experience them personally. Travel Club members exchange stories and provide good information as to where to go, what to avoid and what to do at travel destinations.

25. **Adventure Travel** – Adventure travel takes travel to another level. It can be anywhere, from exploring Patagonia on long wilderness hikes, to seeing an Orangutan preserve in Thailand. You can ride your bicycle for 50 miles/80 kms per day touring Ireland, hike up a mountain, or paddle down some river in New Zealand. On my transatlantic cruise, I met an Australian couple on their way to hike the Camino de Santiago from France through northern Spain. They had traveled all over the world. If they liked a place, they would stay there for weeks. A former nurse and her husband loved to go on Safaris in South Africa. Another couple chased sun and lunar eclipses everywhere. Go on line and search Adventure Travel, you may be surprised.

26. **Gardening** – There is nothing like feeling dirt between your fingers as you plant that seedling. It makes you feel a part of nature making something grow. You watch that seed pop out of the ground and become a beautiful flower. Some people love Bromeliads, others orchids or roses. Growing Bonsai trees can be a real challenge. Join a gardening club. If you grow your own vegetables, you will have pure food for your body to enjoy.

27. **Cooking Clubs** – My best friend loves to cook and bake. She finds that cooking a variety of good tasting dishes is rewarding and a diversion from her day job. The creative process of blending spices and ingredients allows her to relax. Cooking Clubs explore a variety of dishes and styles. They re-define subtleties in flavors that most of us never experienced. You can also go to a Culinary School.

28. **Volunteer Organizations** – If you want another purpose in life, give back to society. Help those in need to get them back on their feet. Being a volunteer for worthy causes can be very rewarding and a good use of your spare time. Philanthropy, if you have the resources, can be an engaging and rewarding endeavor.

29. **Museum Docent** – Some people just love museums. Being a docent and knowing everything about the artist can be a fulfilling volunteer activity.

30. **Dog Walking** – People that love dogs, Love dogs. Did I say love dogs? Help a pet sitter on a part time basis so that she can take a vacation and fill in when she is too busy. You can also get involved in dog rescue or raise puppies for guide dog organizations.

31. **Senior Learning Colleges** – This is a big one. Lifelong Learning is very important for continued brain development. In St Petersburg, Florida, we have ASPEC (Academy of Senior Professionals at Eckerd College), OLLI (Osher Lifelong Learning Institute), USF (University of South Florida) with free noncredit college courses, and the St Petersburg College lifelong learning classes. Most large communities have some form of lifelong learning. My 83 year old sister in Poland

learned how to operate a computer at such a class and has become a virtual traveler and student. You can also check with high schools and libraries for any adult courses being offered.

32. **Continuing Education** – If you are a professional, it's good to keep learning in your field. Personally, I go to as many continuing medical education lectures as I can. My routine involves attending 1- 2 hours of continuing medical education (Grand Rounds) each week. The lectures keep me informed of the newest developments in medicine. They are also a good way to interact with people that have a similar education. The post-seminar lunch conversations, can become intellectually stimulating and lots of fun. As my sister, a former math teacher, said, "I exercise my brain."

33. **Mentoring Programs** – Many new business entrepreneurs and professionals may need mentors to become successful. They could use your expertise to become better in their profession. You will feel better because you have helped someone achieve their dreams. Big Brother, Big Sister and the Scouts are good organizations to help young people flourish.

34. **Volunteering in Animal Shelters** – Help an abandoned or stray animal find a good home. Dog rescue programs, Friends of Strays and the Humane Society always need volunteers.

35. **Hospital Volunteer** – Hospitals need volunteers of all kinds. You can be running the gift shop or assisting nurses and patients. Being a Hospice volunteer can be very rewarding. Get involved and find out what volunteers your local hospital needs.

36. **Religious Organizations** – Places of worship need volunteers to help the community flourish. You can get involved in anything from education, church fairs, or after-school care, to providing meals on wheels for the elderly and sick. Going on mission trips to help the underprivileged improve their lives can be very rewarding.

37. **Special Interest Meetup Groups** – Go online and type in meetup groups in your area. You will be surprised by the large variety of groups that get together.

38. Writers' Groups – If you have always wanted to write a book, find a writers group and learn how the process works. You will benefit from the knowledge of other authors.

39. Inventors' Clubs – We have one in Tampa Bay. Members discuss their ideas, show prototypes, get feedback and learn how to patent and protect their inventions.

40. Car Restoration – For car buffs, restoring an old car is fascinating. You can see a rust bucket turn into a beautiful piece of art that you can show off at car shows. The same holds true for either old boat or motorcycle restorations. I've met Brits restoring old trains through vintage train clubs.

41. Fashion Clubs – An old friend of mine loved to watch fashion and designer shows on television. Get together with like-minded people and follow the latest fashion trends. Your club can travel to fashion shows.

42. Antiquing – Try making the old new again. People love antiques. There is a television show just dedicated to that. There are flea markets and antique fairs all over the place. Someone that I knew spent a lifetime collecting things of value and now he is selling his valuables on line to other collectors.

43. Investor Groups – Investor group meetups are in most retirement areas. Be careful and make hypothetical purchases for an extended period before you start throwing real money into the game. The group meetups are good for learning and discussing investment options.

44. Symphony – If you love classical music, going to the weekly symphony or pops concerts is an enjoyable way to spend Saturday afternoons or evenings. Opera and Ballet are other options.

45. Theatre – Community Theatre exists everywhere. Become an actress, actor, stage hand or just support the theatre company by going to their plays. I love going to see live theatre, either on Broadway or at a local playhouse.

46. Playing in a Band – Many of you were in a high school band. Did you know that there are marching bands for former band members? In St Petersburg, Florida, it's called *The Second Time Arounders Marching Band*. If you played an instrument or were a majorette in high school, find a group of people and jam with them. In Stephenville, Newfoundland, I heard *The Folks on the Bay* a group of fiddlers, guitar players, banjo players and drummers that played a variety of folk and Irish music.

47. **Learning a Musical Instrument** – Learning to play a new musical instrument can be both challenging and rewarding. The dedication and time required can make your brain grow younger. Mastering a musical instrument is as much of an anti-aging activity as dancing or walking.

48. **Choirs or Choral groups** – My mother loved to sing in the church choir. In my area we also have the *Madrigals*, a choral group that sings old English *a cappella* songs in the Madrigal style. If you love to sing, join your church choir or a choral group.

49. **Wine-Tasting** – Wine-tastings are available in wine stores, private clubs and restaurants. If you enjoy fine wines, go and find your perfect dinner wine or wine for special occasions. It's a good way to socialize.

50. **Shuffle Board Clubs** – St Petersburg, Florida, was once world famous for its shuffle board courts. Guess what? Shuffle board is coming back, and the old shuffle board courts are now filled with retirees in the daytime and young people on dates on Friday and Saturday nights.

51. **Sailing Race Official** – This is a niche hobby that few people ever think about. Yacht racing requires people to organize and run the regattas. If you love being on the water, have you ever thought about running sailboat regattas or powerboat-predicted log races?

52. **Flying Clubs** – In Lakeland, Florida, and Oshkosh, Wisconsin, the EAA (Experimental Aircraft Association) has yearly fly-ins. People from all over the world go there to see the latest developments in ultralights, sport planes, gliders and personal aircraft. The daily air shows are spectacular. Last year I saw a jet powered biplane do amazing aerial acrobatics. Local airports all have flying clubs that you can get involved in.

53. **RV Travel – Recreational Vehicles** and retirement go together like peanut butter and jelly. A great portion of this

book was written in my RV traveling in Northeastern Canada and the United States. I met fellow RVers that told me of other places that I may want to visit. One couple that I met had been full time RV-ers for 10 years and saw every part of the US, Alaska and Canada twice. They enjoyed the National Parks and wildlife sanctuaries the most. In mid-January, at the Florida Fairgrounds in Tampa, we have the Florida RV Super-Show, one of the largest in the world. Another huge RV show, The Caravan Salon, takes place in the fall, in Dusseldorf, Germany (www.caravan-salon.com).

I met an American couple, who for the past 15 years, have lived all over western and eastern Europe. They come back to the States on a cruise ship every couple of years in the fall. They rent an apartment and a car in Sarasota, Florida, for 6 months, and then take another cruise ship back to Europe in the spring. There are many RV travel clubs you can join, as well as caravans that do all the planning for you. Go online and read the blogs of people traveling in RVs.

54. **Boating/Cruising Clubs** – Boat owners like to get together at various yacht clubs and marinas, socialize and have dinner. It's a good way to meet other boaters and see the area. You can go cruise either in a power boat or a sailboat. Some cruising clubs are just for Sailboats and others have both sail and power. There are also online meet-up boat clubs.

55. **Ship Cruising** – The cruise industry just keeps on growing with cruises being offered all over the world. Many people like cruising because you get to see different parts of the world in a floating hotel. Just remember to walk those decks, or go to the fitness classes on board, to maintain your weight and to stay in shape. The relocation cruises have a very high percentage of retirees on them from all over the world. What interests me is talking to all those fascinating people, to discover what they did in their careers, and what their current interests in retirement are. If you sit with random people at large tables, you will learn a lot about people's interests, which in turn may spur on your interests.

This morning I sat with Jan, a 70 year old molecular biophysicist who dove 20,000 feet under the ocean in a research submarine studying tube worms living by volcanic vents. She spends over 180 days a year cruising in ships, which includes around the world cruises. If you like quiet cruising, consider going on a cargo ship with passenger cabins. Some people even live full time on cruise ships. Food, entertainment, room service, and social interaction – sounds like a winning combination to me.

56. **Aerobics Classes** – Fitness clubs and the YMCA offer these popular classes regularly. From the morning stretch to Zumba to body pump aerobics, it's a good way to stay in shape and be motivated by your fellow participants.

57. **Swimming** – Swimming is one of the best exercises you can have. Most retirement communities have pools. A daily swim can make you feel refreshed and all limbered up. You could join a local swimming club.

58. **Learning Another Language** – You have always wanted to learn German, Italian, French, Chinese or Spanish, haven't you? If you really want your brain to grow, learn another language in retirement. For a real challenge, try Polish.

59. **Cultural Immersion in Another Society** – What better way is there to learn about another society than actually living there for a few months? You experience their food, entertainment, culture and how they think. It's a good way to develop an appreciation for other cultures and a different perspective.

60. **Woodworking** – Having a small woodworking workshop in your home can be very relaxing and creative. There are woodworking clubs that have machines that you can use for making your creative furniture, rocking chair or baby crib projects.

61. **Model Plane Flying** – If you can't get the big plane, get the small plane and fly it at a local model plane club. One of my neighbors had two model jet planes in his garage that flew 400 miles (643 kilometers) per hour.

62. **Model Sailboat Racing Club** – Radio-controlled sailboat racing is just as competitive as racing big sailboats. The boat class size is standardized and the wind is the same for everyone.

63. **Dining Out** – If you like to sample different restaurants, dining out is a good way to spend time with your spouse or friends. Some people just love the subtleties of foods and wines. You could join an epicurean club along with a wine club to develop your taste buds. Small portions along with exercise are essential if you love food.

64. **Bowling League** – Bowling is a good way to get involved in a group activity or to just have fun with your loved ones and friends. There are bowling leagues everywhere.

65. **Sporting Events** – Many retirees like going to sporting events. Baseball, hockey, football, soccer and basketball are popular spectator events. The afternoon baseball games are filled with retirees having a great time. Hot dogs and Cracker Jack are just as popular now as they were 75 years ago.

66. **Skiing** – One of my friends is 84 years old and skis like a teenager. Tampa Bay has one of the largest ski clubs in the country comprising many northerners who retired here and still like to ski. There are trips offered all over the world.

67. **Parachuting** – Certain people like the thrill of jumping out of an airplane at least once in their lifetime. I was quite surprised, on a recent cruise, by how many people raised their hands when the comedian asked them if they ever went parachuting.

68. **Experimental Aircraft Building** – A friend of mine built an ultra-light airplane in his garage that he fitted with pontoons. The EAA (The Experimental Aircraft Association) has a large variety of planes at their shows.

69. **Homemade Racing Boats** - Friends of mine built small eight-foot race boats that competed with highly tuned ten-horsepower engines on local lakes. There is a large variety of classes of small boats you can race, just like there is in car racing.

70. **Car Racing** – If you love speed, watching car racing can be an exciting sport to follow. In St Petersburg the St Pete Grand Prix is an annual event. It is an open wheel Indy car race similar

to the Formula 1. People from all over the world come to watch this event and it is televised globally. Barcelona, Spain, and other major cities in the world have Grand Prix races. By going to those events you will get to explore places you haven't visited.

71. **Model Building** – Model building is an art form that requires a great deal of attention to detail. You may enjoy the process of starting with nothing and creating a beautiful scale model sailing ship or plane. Model building, just like jewelry making, is relaxing to a lot of people.

73 **Bird Watching** – Bird-watching is probably one thing you never thought of. There is a whole group of people (birders) that communicate with each other constantly on the internet about rare species of birds that they have seen. They will drive hundreds of miles to find a rare bird that someone has spotted. I have run into them many times at nature preserves carrying large cameras with monopods so that they can take just the right photo of that exotic bird. They will post that photo on the internet for other birders. Some people also like to record bird songs with high quality portable audio recorders. Before my last cruise, I recorded bird songs that I heard every morning where I live. Listening to their recorded singing voices makes my cruise ship cabin feel more like home. Birders will even spend a year traveling to see how many birds they can spot in one year.

At breakfast on my recent transatlantic cruise, a 79 year old man from Sun City Center, Florida, told me that he and his wife had been long-time birders. They told me of going birding to South Africa, spending a month in Tasmania, the Texas birding festival, the Rio Grande valley and of bird migratory patterns. They volunteer at wildlife refuges where they are able to stay free in their RV in exchange for working three days per week at the refuge. After listening to all their stories about where they traveled in their RV for 16 years, and their birding expeditions, it made me realize that the world is your canvas and it is up to you to find out what to put on it.

74. Ham Radio Clubs – One of my rollerblading buddies is actively involved in both a ham radio network and an emergency response communication organization. You would be surprised just how many people are interested in ham radios. On my cruise, I met a German man talking about his ham radio, and across the table from him was an Australian doing the same thing. They instantly hit it off talking about their equipment and the people they talked to all over the world. Being a ham radio operator, you develop friends in distant lands that you can go and visit

75. Short Film Production - is an art form that few people think of. At the Wanee Music Festival in northern Florida, between a band change, I interviewed a man who was a retired builder. When I asked him what he did for fun in retirement, he told me that he teaches photography at the art institute, and he has also won an award for short film production. He likes the creativity of writing and putting a short film together. He said that he was creative as a builder and now in short film production. Photography allowed him to stay creative also.

76. Treasure Hunting Metal Detection. – One of my bicycle group members belongs to a ring finder club. People call them up if they lost a ring on the beach and they will locate it for them.

77. Working Part Time - I knew a lady that retired to Florida with her engineer husband. In retirement, she decided to become a real estate agent specializing in high rise buildings near where she lived. She moved from a 5 bedroom home up north to a spacious one-bedroom condo downtown. When I asked her why she made such a drastic change, she said that she had lots of kids and relatives, and she did not want to be a bed and breakfast for everyone coming down in the winter to visit. A beautiful Hilton hotel was just down the street so they could easily see each other as often they wanted. The 1,050 square foot, one bedroom, condo was easy to take care of and big enough for both of them. To keep herself occupied, she thought that being a realtor and meeting all kinds of interesting people moving to Florida would be a lot of fun. She absolutely loved her retirement job. She enjoyed being socially engaged, talking to new people, and also making some money at the same time. Her husband was happy just playing baseball, monitoring their investments and going to cultural events. He was glad that she found something fulfilling to do in retirement. The arrangement worked for both of them.

On my transatlantic voyage at the breakfast table I met Andy. The man looked like he was 68 years old. He told me, "As a human species we were bred to work," and "What else can you do in an 8 hour day?" He had worked in manufacturing as a mechanical engineer, lived in St Petersburg, Florida, Lake Tahoe, Nevada, Arizona, and now lives in Las Vegas, Nevada, selling real estate part time. He likes to work, "I drive around in my golf cart showing people plots of land and now and then they write me a check. Life is good. I am 87 years old." He was an amazing man to talk to, fit, sharp, and full of energy. I couldn't believe he was 87, he was in such good shape.

New research at the university in Melbourne, Australia, showed that working 25-30 hours per week sharpens your cognitive skills. The last chapter of this book, *The Healthy Mind Active, Happy, and Stress Free*, explores memory enhancement in more detail.

One day, on a morning walk, I saw an older gentleman in his late 70s carefully masking the decorative shutters on a six unit apartment building. I asked him, "Do you own this building?" He said, "Yes, I do." "Do you want to sell it?" He stood there and thought, and shook his head, "No." He then added, "Then I would have nothing to do." He felt that he needed to get out and do something on a regular basis, to stay active. It probably kept him in a better mood, also, and gave him a reason to get out of the house. There are, certainly, many ways to work part-time.

78. Spending Time with Grandchildren – In Malaga, Spain, I met an energetic 75 year old lady from Minnesota. During our lunch conversation with both her and her husband, she told me that helping raise her grandchildren kept her mind young. She would periodically go and help her daughters with their children. Since she has 6 grandchildren of different ages, keeping up with them all keeps her very busy. She feels that she has a close relationship with all her grandkids. For 10 years, they had a winter home in Florida where her kids and grandkids would come down to visit. She could instil her values, and also her faith in God, on the grandkids. She played soccer and baseball and all the things kids like to do. She felt that spending a lot of time with those young kids kept her mentally sharp. She also had to be in good physical shape to keep up with them. In the end, it makes you realize that family is the most important thing in life.

CHAPTER 3

Clean Out/Detoxify Your Body

Imagine living in a house for forty, fifty, sixty, or seventy years. How much junk do you accumulate? Are you running out of storage space? Can you find anything you want at a moment's notice? Do you buy things over, and over, and over again because you forgot where you put them?

Furthermore, your neighbors periodically added things to your storage area. You had no idea what they were adding. They would just stop by and plop things here and there, filling up your house. They didn't come uninvited. You invited them in, and they always brought something with them and left it somewhere in your house.

Sounds farfetched, doesn't it?

"Wait a minute," you say. "I'd never invite neighbors who would bring something to my house, clutter up my home, and then continue filling it up." Most logical people wouldn't, would they? However, what if you didn't know that these neighbors were bringing things in and cluttering up your house? You would continue to invite them because you liked having them over. They're nice, friendly, fun to chat with. They're great company. You have a laugh or two. Life is merry and jolly.

Over time, your house (or your body) becomes so cluttered that you cannot live in it anymore and it starts to self-destruct. Those friendly neighbors are the foods that you eat, and the things they clutter your house up with are the chemicals, additives and preservatives in the food.

We have no idea what's in our food, the things we touch, what's in the air we breathe, or in the water we drink. Do we?

All of us get thermal printed receipts from stores every day. Did you know that the thermal paper is coated with BPA (Bisphenol A) or the chemically related BPS and BPF? These chemicals are absorbed through the skin on our fingers and react with our hormonal system. They are endocrine disrupters that are of special concern to women of child bearing age, pregnant or nursing, teenagers and even the elderly. These chemicals can imitate our bodies' own hormones and have undesirable consequences. According to studies done in Europe and Japan, they apparently mimic estrogen and influence how cells respond to natural estrogens. In animal studies, BPA was linked to obesity, cancer and reproductive problems. In humans, BPA has been associated with increased risk of diabetes and heart disease.

Isn't it sad that something as minuscule as a thermal store receipt may be harmful to us? How about the chemical compounds released by all the plastic containers that we microwave in? It would be safer not to touch those receipts, and learn to microwave in glass or lead free ceramic containers. A PhD friend of mine only uses stainless water bottles on his bicycle to prevent possible plastic leaching of chemicals. Another doctor friend of mine has the receipts put in the grocery bag so that she doesn't have to touch them.

Our hormones are being replaced by unnatural chemicals that mimic hormones but do not do the same thing. To illustrate the danger that certain chemicals have on our finely tuned "dance of the hormones" think of locks and keys. Each lock has a specific key that unlocks it. Some keys can fit into several keyholes but they may not unlock all the doors. A key may be made from a similar blank, but the pattern of ridges on the key is different so it may fit in a lock but not open the door. These synthetic chemicals are like the blank keys that may fit in the lock but cannot open the door.

If a lock has a key in it that doesn't open the door can the correct key be inserted on top of that key to open that door? No, it cannot. Your room stays locked and you can't do anything with what's inside that door. If it's a car, you can't drive the car. If you are a mechanic, you cannot unlock your tool box to repair a car. If it's your pantry, you cannot go in and get the ingredients to cook or bake, can you?

Maybe that's why young ladies cannot get pregnant because the keyholes are full of useless synthetic estrogen keys? Maybe that's why we get cancer, because the keyholes have blank keys in them and our immune repair system keys cannot get in and fix our bodies.

Food for Thought: It took millions of years of evolution for our bodies to adapt to the foods we eat. Plants and other food sources evolved with us at the same pace, and our bodies learned how to use them for fuel and adapt to them. Suddenly, in the 21st century, we have thousands of chemicals thrown at us that we have not had time to adapt to, nor been able to detoxify. How can we expect our immune system to adapt to so many synthetic products in our food chain in such a short time? It is all too fast and very dangerous. Our foods have become our poisons. Think about this for a while.

Trans-fatty Acids and Hydrogenated Oils: In the late 1990s I saw a report about trans-fatty acids on prime time national news. The headline was, effectively, "The Fats You Eat May Be Killing You". It was a catchy headline, so I hung around listening to the main report, and it was about trans-fatty acids and hydrogenated oils. These are used throughout the processed food industry to preserve flavors in food and keep it from spoiling. Now, the experts are saying that these trans-fatty acids may be clogging your arteries and might be one of the leading causes of the high incidences of cardiovascular disease and arteriosclerosis.

See, these things are not really natural, so the body has no effective way of eliminating them or dealing with them. As we were developing through the millions of years, our bodies developed to accommodate common things found in nature: animal fats, vegetables, proteins, carbohydrates, trace minerals, vitamins, and so forth. Bodies did not evolve to process the hundred thousand chemicals we are exposed to on a continuous basis. Many of these things are man-made.

The FDA has finally banned the use of trans-fatty acids, and it is to go into effect in 2018. It took a lawsuit and overwhelming evidence for them to act. Why did it take so long?

What about white bread? Is the FDA finally going to do something about it? You may wonder what I am talking about. In order to make white bread the grain has to be bleached with either chlorine or other chemicals. This bleaching process destroys many naturally occurring vitamins and nutrients and potentially adds alloxan, a byproduct of the bleaching process. Alloxan is used in laboratory animals to induce diabetes. The bleaching process also allows more sugar to be added to the bread. With the huge rise of diabetes in this country, does eating bleached white bread make sense? The use of chlorine, bromates, and peroxides in food is banned in the European Union.

If you think that eating bleached bread is bad, how about eating plastic. A plastic material called azodicarbonamide (ADA) has been reported to be in 500 foods. It makes bread and pastries spongy; that's why it is also used in flip flops and exercise mats. The thought of eating my flip flops makes me cringe.

Have you ever thought about coffee? Most of us drink this beverage every morning. Do you know whether the coffee beans have been sprayed with pesticides? Did you know that coffee plants have up to 250 pounds of pesticides per acre sprayed on them? We may be grinding and boiling those pesticides right into our bodies. True, there may be some high-end, mountain-grown coffee beans out there that pesticide machines can't reach, but most of us are totally unaware which beans are pesticide-free, since most are imported. Check to see if the coffee is certified organic, labeled sustainable, or grown traditionally. Coffee is cardio-protective and helps reduce the incidence of type 2 diabetes according to the newest research. Two to five cups of coffee appear to be OK according to the new US dietary guidelines.

The fruits and vegetables we eat are all sprayed to prevent bugs and fungi from eating them. What effect are those pesticides having on our bodies? Even if we wash our fruits and vegetables thoroughly the small quantities absorbed through their skins may still be enough to cause chronic diseases from 10 to 40 years later because they slowly accumulate in our system. As the saying goes, "Buyer beware," because the food that we consume may slowly be destroying us, and specific food that we fail to consume (example?), may be required to protect us from those adulterated food toxins.

Over the last fifty to sixty years, big business, primarily the food and biochemical industries, have figured out how to make things taste good, look good and last forever. They also created **GMOs** – genetically modified organisms. In their quest for economic gain, they didn't take into consideration the long term effects of these chemical substances and altered genes on our health. It's all about yield per acre (hectare), money and profit.

Due to our industrialized society, millions of tons of toxic waste are created. However, there is nowhere to put it. So, the government allows this toxic waste residue, created from large manufacturing companies and smouldering plants, to be ground up, mixed into fertilizers, and spread upon our soil. These toxins are absorbed by the plants along with the fertilizer, passed on through the food chain, and we, as the ultimate consumers of the food chain, absorb them in our bodies. Pressure-treated wood has enough toxins in it, such as arsenic, to be considered a hazard. Did you know that it was excluded from the hazardous waste law? (WAC 173-303-071)

You had no idea they were doing that, did you? Very few people do, just as you had no idea of the risks that accompany what you ingest into your system. A sludge-infested body is more susceptible to a variety of ailments.

This living house of yours has existed for forty to eighty years. That's a long time for junk to accumulate and clog up your biological system. You invite the junk through the foods you eat. Probably the most recognizable form of clogging is cardiovascular disease. Years and years of accumulation of bad, processed, and genetically altered fats combined with other toxic elements in our food, air, and environment slowly clog up the system. Eventually, the system breaks down and develops obstruction of the blood supply to major organs.

When that obstruction occurs in the heart, we get restriction of blood flow, oxygenation and nutrients to the heart muscle causing heart stress. If enough damage occurs, the heart attack we get leads to total heart failure and our demise.

Modern medicine's solution to that problem is to insert a stent or a bypass of two to three inches of a blood vessel from a vein grafted from your leg. That vein is not as strong as the original vessel it replaces and it might eventually also clog up.

The bypass procedure is nothing more than an expensive Band-Aid for an emergency treatment. It does not cure the disease. It does make people feel better and it does increase blood supply to certain sections of the heart for a limited time.

Did you ever ask yourself, "What about the other seventy- five million miles of blood vessels that I have in my body? What's happening to them and the rest of my organ systems and my brain? Are they getting enough blood supply and nutrition?"

The answer is obvious. If it is obstructing your heart, it is obstructing the rest of your system.

How about the clogging of less obvious systems, which occurs in Alzheimer's disease or other chronic ailments, that can eventually lead to abnormal cell functions and ultimately our death. In Alzheimer's disease, researchers have found higher concentrations of aluminum, as well as a sludge-type material, beta amyloid, the residue of dead nerve cells, neurofibrillary tangles, and abnormal accumulation of Tau protein and neuro inflammation.

This sludge-type material eventually clogs up the cell mechanisms so the nerve cells cannot communicate and function properly. After a while, they become so inundated with the garbage that has been deposited over the years they die.

As neurons die, you gradually lose the ability to think. How sad, spending a lifetime achieving goals, being active, relishing your children and grandchildren, and not to be able to enjoy your old age. By the way, what do you have when you get older? You have your memories. When your memories are gone, as in former president Ronald Reagan's case, you can't even enjoy your past achievements in old age. A part of your life has been robbed.

What about cancer, and other chronic degenerative conditions?

Cancer is a failure of your body to regulate itself, a failure in the immune system. It's going back to the same mechanism that caused your cardiovascular disease, caused your Alzheimer's disease, and causes a lot of other chronic conditions. It is a sludging-up of your system with junk breaking down your automatic repair processes. It is a failure of your immune system to keep you healthy. . It cannot repair itself properly and the cells may continue to replicate themselves unchecked until they kill you.

The checks and balances are lost because there is so much junk built up in your system. The more chemicals you inject through processed foods and additives, the greater your chances of developing a chronic disease that your body can't handle because there is too much sludge clogging up your natural reparative mechanisms.

The modern agricultural food business, including the fast- food industry, has produced food that is loaded with sugar and devoid of essential nutrients, vitamins and minerals, and loaded with chemical additives, preservatives, and unnatural fats. More than half of the United States population is either overweight or obese, and at the same time nutritionally starved.

This greed for profit in our food industry has created a time-bomb in our population that will eventually lead to a slew of chronic degenerative diseases and which will make the quality of our lives miserable.

There is a remedy: Clean out the body and give it pure and nutrient-laden foods, necessary supplements, and adequate amounts of pure, clean, unadulterated water. Water is essential for cleansing our body, increasing the function of our kidneys, and normalizing our cellular fluids, both intra- and extracellular. You want to give your liver, the main detoxifying organ, a rest.

Detoxification is the removal of toxic substances from our body. It is primarily done by the liver, but other organs such as the kidneys, the lymph system, skin and lungs also act as detoxifiers. You have heard of alcohol detox, drug detox, poison antidotes, narcotics overdose antidotes and dialysis. Dialysis is detoxification because your kidneys are not doing their job anymore filtering out toxins. If your liver fails, you need a transplant. For prescription drug detoxification there is a detox program called the Xenobiotic Mechanism, which involves a series of oxidase reactions to neutralize the drug. There is detoxification going on all the time in your body. So, what can you do to help that process along?

The first thing you do is limit your invitations to the neighbors visiting your living-house, those friendly, happy go lucky elements that are depositing junk all over the place and clogging it up to the point where things start breaking down. Yes, I know. Fatty foods, fries, greasy chicken, processed foods, all kinds of snack food, and ready-to-

John P. Lenhart M.D.

eat meals are things you enjoy. Of course they are. They are engineered to taste good, look good, and smell good. They are not necessarily engineered to be healthy.

You may enjoy eating them, but consider the long-term consequences. The first thing you need to do is to limit what you take in. This will be discussed in more detail in a later chapter.

The next thing you have to do, as the title of this chapter says, is clean your system out. Detoxify yourself. You see, once your body gets rid of a large portion of the stored toxins and sludge that was accumulated over a long period of time, it will be more organized. The biological processes will work better, the chemical interactions, digestion, repair mechanisms will all function optimally. An optimized system will decrease your chances of developing chronic debilitating diseases, such as adult onset diabetes, cancer, cardiovascular disease, Alzheimer's disease, and so on. If your body works at peak efficiency, there is less chance of biological breakdown, which causes a lot of these disease processes. The less stress you put on the system, the better it will work. Just think of work stress, emotional stress, and financial stress. If there is enough stress on the system, eventually something has to give. You want to limit your chemical stress, psychological stress and environmental stress as much as possible to prevent that break down.

There are numerous ways one can detoxify oneself. One of the oldest ways of detoxification is sweating. It is a tradition that started in Europe, Turkey, and the Middle East where people used saunas to induce perspiration. The theory was that by sweating, toxins could be eliminated through the skin's pores and this allowed the body to purify itself. Sweating is an effective way to rid the body of excess waste through your skin.

The largest organ in our body is our skin. It is very efficient in eliminating excess waste and fluids from the body. Without skin, we would die. A good example is people whose skin has been severely burned over large portions of their bodies. With so much of their skin damaged, they easily succumb to infections and may die.

Skin is also a semi-permeable membrane. Certain substances pass right through it. Therefore, external toxins we touch, or are exposed to in the air, are absorbed by our skin and can poison us slowly. Medications, also, are now given through the skin through patches and creams.

Just as the skin absorbs toxins, the skin can excrete toxins. Taking saunas or steam baths has been a popular method of detoxification throughout the centuries and is currently used extensively throughout the world. Around the world, people go to spas so that they can stay healthy.

Another way of obtaining similar benefits is by exercising to the point where you sweat. These kinds of exercise and their duration, will be addressed in a later chapter.

Unlike exercising to produce sweat, sauna sweating requires no effort. You just sit there and let your metabolism do the work. The body tries to cool itself because of the excess heat, and it does that by perspiring. As the body perspires, toxins are released. Drinking eight to ten glasses of pure water per day is a simple way to clean out your system and help you sweat.

There are a number of herbal teas that have been used for detoxification as well. You can find many of them in the health stores. Ginseng is one of the most common detoxification agents. Chamomile tea, used in Europe quite a bit, is another. Ginkgo biloba has also become popular as has Essiac tea.

Herbal teas are even being used to pass drug tests. If you look on the Internet, you'll find several companies that have various herbal tea products that cause you to urinate and detoxify any drug residue left in your body, allowing people to pass drug tests. As noted in the above examples, herbs are potent detoxifying agents.

For a zinger of a detoxifying tea, you may try the Garlic – Ginger tea. It consists of a bulb of crushed garlic, a thinly sliced lemon, a handful of thinly sliced ginger, a pinch or two of turmeric, cayenne pepper and honey. The garlic, ginger and turmeric are boiled for an hour in about a liter or quart of water. After boiling add the sliced lemon and a pinch of cayenne pepper (do not touch the pepper with your fingers or rub your eyes) and let it sit 20min. You can add some more water, and then strain the contents for the tea. Add honey, while hot, 1-2 teaspoons before drinking. You can refrigerate and reheat the tea adding honey each time before drinking. You may be surprised how you feel afterwards. You may catch fewer colds in the flu season, or when flying in planes.

On our web site happylifehealthyaging.com we will have various detoxification methods that have been used by others.

One form of detoxification and cleansing that is often ignored is fasting. Our bodies were designed to have periods of starvation. To encounter periods of starvation is part of our nutritional cycle. Through the thousands of years of human development, there has never existed a period of time where food was as plentiful as it is today. . Therefore, the body has adapted to storing as many nutrients as possible in our fat cells when there is plenty, and to utilize those nutrients in periods of food deficiency.

This cycle of feast and famine was normal in our human evolutionary development. It also played an important component in ridding our bodies of unnecessary toxins that developed in the plentiful cycle. However, with the abundance and excess of food, this normal cleansing phase has not had a chance to kick in, and we have continuously stored toxins absorbed through our food chain, and through our skin and lungs, without a chance to refresh ourselves.

Fasting has been used throughout the centuries as a method to purify the body. There are numerous biblical references to fasting dating back thousands of years. Many religions use fasting as a purification before their major holidays. It was not just for self-sacrifice that fasting was used. Fasting was recognized as a means of cleansing the body of impurities.

A number of years ago, while I was studying for my first doctorate, I developed an interest in fasting and I read a well-documented, out-of-print book on fasting. The book was written before World War Two and broke down, specifically, the body's physiological responses to fasting.

When the body is not getting external energy from proteins, carbohydrates, or fats, it has to look internally for reserves. This internal approach mobilizes biochemical processes and chemical reactions that are not normally used.

This triggering of chemical reactions, which forces the body to utilize glycogen, fat, and even protein stores of fuel, mobilizes some of the stored impurities embedded in our fat cells. As the fat is burned for fuel, some of those impurities are excreted through the urinary system and skin.

Periodic fasts of one to three days are used routinely in European countries as cleansing mechanisms, which allow the body's unused biochemical processes to function, thereby providing us with alternative sources of fuel. When I did my last fast of 2.5 days, I drank sparkling water and occasionally added 1-2 oz. of Gatorade or orange juice for electrolytes and flavor. I lost 7 lbs. and felt great. During my fast I walked 3 hours the second day and kept hydrated. When I started to eat, it was only a small amount of food and mostly fruits and vegetables with some protein. Your stomach shrinks so you feel full right away. Two days after fasting, I had a lot of energy without the desire to eat a lot of food.

Intermittent fasting has become the new fast. Researchers at several universities have started to study the effects of intermittent fasting on our physiology by doing controlled, before and after, blood work studies. The most popular intermittent fast is the 5:2 fast. For five days you eat normally, and for 2 days you reduce your calorie intake to 600 calories if you are a man, and 500 calories if you are a woman. The theory behind this intermittent fast is that it is protein sparing. You burn primarily glycogen and fat instead of muscle for energy.

Always ask your doctor if your health condition is able to tolerate a fast. With the rampant progress of diabetes and other health conditions around us, you may not be able to tolerate even an intermittent fast.

It is important to remember that copious amounts of water are necessary when one undergoes a fasting program since water is a key ingredient in many of the biochemical reactions to burn body stores of fuel.

I generally recommend at least one-half to one gallon (2.2 to 3 plus liters) of water per day to help boost metabolism. In my practice I have seen mild bladder infections clear up with a gallon of water a day and some cranberry juice mixed in. Newer scientific research has shown that cranberry juice helps prevent bacteria from adhering to the bladder wall therefore reducing the incidence of infections. The studies did not find, however, that once an infection has established itself, cranberry juice could get rid of it, therefore making antibiotic drugs a necessity.

We can self-detoxify by flushing out our systems with pure, osmotically-filtered, or distilled water in adequate amounts. We can assist the body in flushing itself on a daily basis, giving a continuous cleansing, the same way that daily bowel movements move digested waste out of our systems so that we don't absorb the harmful chemicals that are collecting in our guts. Colonoscopies have become routine and help detect early colon cancers. They are recommended to be done by age 50 and every 10 years thereafter. Colon cancer is one of the few preventable cancers if detected in the pre-cancerous stage by a colonoscopy.

Talking about our gut leads us to another commonly used form of detoxification, colonic irrigation. Colonics do not sound pleasant. As a matter of fact, they sound repulsive. However, Fleet enemas have been a long-standing part of medical procedures for both constipation and cleansing the gut of fecal toxins that have been accumulating. A colonic is a deeper form of intestinal cleansing. The practitioner performing the procedure must be a licensed and certified health care provider that uses sterile equipment, so that there is no cross contamination from others. Probiotics may be a good idea afterwards to make sure you have adequate beneficial bacteria in your gut.

Chronic constipation, or improper bowel motility, can lead to chronic diseases. At times, inadequate intestinal motility to eliminate impacted particles, or feces, can create little pockets and cause craters leading to, you guessed it, colon cancer, polyps, or overall illness, as the byproducts of digestion can actually be toxic. The indoles and skatols that are produced, as well as other chemicals, are harmful to the body. A colonic is a process whereby you lie on your side, draped, and a sterile canula is inserted into your rectum. Warm water is circulated through your bowels and extracted. Any impacted or stagnant material is flushed out and eliminated, leaving you with a clean gut. It's not as awful as it sounds and is not painful. The reason that I informed you of colonics is because few people have heard of them. If you have impaction problems, colonics are an option to consider. Colonoscopy preps are another.

Other enemas have also been used to detoxify the gut. The purpose of informing you about gut cleansing is to make you aware that the intestinal system can be a source of auto-intoxication and, therefore, needs to be regularly cleaned out. Regular bowel movements are very important. Meat, putrefied in the gut, produces a lot of toxins. Consuming prunes enhances bowel motility as do other forms of roughage.

The last topic I want to talk about regarding "cleaning it out," or detoxification, is chelation therapy. The theory of chelation was invented in Europe at the turn of the twentieth century. As a matter of fact, Dr. Alfred Werner, a German-Swiss scientist, won a Nobel Prize in 1913 for inventing chelation. The German chemical industry had a heck of a time removing impurities from their chemicals, especially the dye industry. They had difficulty getting a pure color because of the calcium deposits, as well as other metal and mineral deposits, that crept into their chemicals. They used Dr. Werner's invention to find the impurities and remove them from their substances so that they would have the pure chemicals that they needed.

Chelation uses a synthetic amino acid, EDTA (ethylene diamine tetra-acetic acid), to bind toxic metals in a heterocyclic ring, a fancy term meaning it encircles the object and forces it to bind to it. In humans, once the toxic metal or mineral is bound, you pee it out. It's simple and effective.

Chelation is used in many of our household goods. One of the most common is mayonnaise. EDTA keeps mayonnaise from going rancid by preventing oxidation, which causes rancidity. By using EDTA, the free radicals cannot destroy the mayonnaise as easily, thereby keeping it fresh. Otherwise, it would spoil within a matter of days. EDTA is a potent antioxidant.

Chelation is also used in shower cleaners. Look at some of the major brands and you will see EDTA as one of the ingredients. It binds the shower scum and helps remove it from your shower walls.

In humans, chelation was first used in the 1950s for people suffering from lead poisoning, as in the battery plants of Detroit, Michigan. Dr. Norman Clark, at Providence Hospital in Detroit, used chelation for the first time to detoxify heavy metals from workers who were exposed to lead and who suffered from numerous neurological conditions due to lead toxicity. After receiving intravenous chelation, the workers got well and their neurological conditions improved.

When Dr. Clark reported his beneficial effects with battery plant workers, chelation caught on for the treatment of heavy-metal poisoning. The U.S. Government started using it to treat painters who painted the bottoms of ships with lead paint. Many ship painters developed severe neurological problems due to heavy-metal toxicity. With chelation therapy, those patients also got better.

As chelation started to be used more and more for toxic metal poisoning (it is still the treatment of choice for children with toxicity from lead paint), doctors started noticing other beneficial effects they had not expected. One of the most prominent was circulatory effects. Patients who had symptoms of arteriosclerotic disease, such as chest pain, intermittent claudication, decreased energy, and so forth, improved and reported fewer chest pains, increased ability to walk and increased energy.

Because of those observations, doctors started using chelation for circulatory problems. Currently, over a million people have received chelation therapy for all kinds of conditions ranging from ulcerations and gangrene of the feet due to diabetes, neuropathy, impaired circulation in the legs, heart and brain, memory loss, decreased energy, and heavy metal toxicity, and also as a preventative measure. I have noticed remarkable results in a lot of my patients who have had chelation therapy at the chelation medical centers.

It appears that when the toxins in our food chain and our environment that have been impeding our body chemical repair and regulatory cycles, are removed, the body functions better. I have seen patients' memory improve. After chelation therapy, patients who had to write sticky notes all over the place to remember things to do, no longer needed those reminders. I have seen patients' diabetic neuropathy improve. I have seen ulcerations improve. Notably, I see a marked increase in energy in a lot of my patients and a willingness to do more and be active in life, even into their old age. One of the more remarkable things I have seen is that patients, even those who have had a stroke, become more alert in terms of their environment. They develop an interest in things, whereas before, they were content to do very little. These are anecdotal findings, reported by relatives that have not been scientifically tested, but nevertheless are worth mentioning.

Chelation therapy is received intravenously. In my chelation centers, patients reclined in comfortable chairs and could read, nap, eat, drink or chat with other patients, while the infusion flowed into their veins.

Chelation therapy is not only the intravenous administration of a synthetic amino acid, EDTA, it also involves administration of certain vitamins concurrently. Patients receive B vitamins, as well as vitamin C, in their drip and are given multiple minerals and multivitamins to supplement any trace elements that are lost but are necessary to the body. Patients are also instructed in dietary changes, as well as exercise regimens to go along with their chelation therapy.

Taking all of that into consideration, not all patients follow the recommendations. Yet, even those who get only the intravenous chelation drip have had remarkable improvements based upon my clinical observations. Numerous other studies have concurred with these observations. Some of those studies will be referenced later in this book.

Since the first edition of this book was written in 2000, a great deal of research has been done on chelation therapy. The National Center for Complementary and Alternative Medicine, a division of the NIH (National Institute of Health), began a Trial to Assess Chelation Therapy (TACT) in 2003 due to pressure from patients and from physicians administering chelation. The trial was to study the validity of chelation for treating conditions other than heavy metal poisoning. The trial was also supported by the American College of Cardiology. Alternative-minded physicians who were certified to administer chelation therapy by ACAM (the American College for the Advancement of Medicine), were observing a variety of benefits in their patients that needed to be investigated further, on a controlled basis.

The study started in 2003 with final results being published November 2012, long after the first edition of this book was published. The authors concluded that disodium EDTA chelation "modestly" reduced the risk of adverse cardiovascular outcomes among stable patients with a history of myocardial infarction. The study also showed a "marked" reduction in cardiovascular events in diabetic patients treated with EDTA chelation. An editorial published in the *Journal of the American Medical Association*(*JAMA*) said that "the study findings may provide novel hypotheses that merit further evaluation to help understand the pathophysiology of secondary prevention of vascular disease."

The surprise for me was the *JAMA* editorial, since there had been so much criticism in the past, of chelation for conditions other than heavy metal toxicity. The words "marked" reduction in cardiovascular events in diabetics were significant to me, since I found peripheral small vessel benefits in my patients where the tingling in their feet disappeared and normal color returned. These were incidental benefits that patients told me about, and they have not been specifically studied in a controlled trial. Patients undergoing EDTA chelation therapy are also advised to follow healthy lifestyle choices such as avoiding saturated fats, eating a lot of fruits and vegetables, increasing exercise and maintaining proper weight.

Use your own judgement and do your own research, since there are differences of opinion regarding this treatment for conditions other than heavy metal poisoning. I included chelation therapy in the detoxifying chapter because it does detoxify and everyone agrees on that. Most doctors have limited knowledge about the benefits of chelation or about this major study.

So, let's tie all this together. I began this chapter with a house that became cluttered with people you invited in, who kept dropping things off and storing them, and you had no idea that they were doing that. These people (friendly foods) inadvertently gave you a fatal disease through the unnatural additives they deposited in your body.

We frequently eat foods in restaurants where the food was cooked in aluminum pans and the aluminum may have been absorbed into the food and eventually deposited into our brains and other tissues. As well, we are finding that there are thousands of chemicals, hormones, antibiotics and additives added to our food. They make food grow faster, look good, and last longer. We inadvertently eat and store these chemicals in our house, our body.

We invite that food into our bodies (as we invite our friends into our house) because it looks good, is pleasant, gives us a good time, and we enjoy looking at, smelling and eating it. However, all of the adulterated foods in our food chain are slowly toxifying us.

The chemical and toxic metal load that is placed upon us gradually wears down our immune systems to the point where our resistance is very low and any abnormal stressor to our systems can set off a chronic degenerative condition. Did you ever ask yourself, with all the miracles of medicine, why is cardiovascular disease the number one killer and cancer the number two killer in the United States?

All of these conditions are self-induced by things we voluntarily store in our bodies, such as cancer-forming chemicals from cigarette smoking, or even artificial sweeteners. As well, we don't know the long-term effects on our bodies through involuntary storage of chemicals from all the processed food we eat on a daily basis.

When was the last time you read the labels of all the foods you eat? Do you know what all the chemical names are that are on those labels? Do you know what they are used for? Do you know how they are stored in the body, or excreted from the body? Do you know what secondary reactions they may have to impede our body from working properly? You don't.

You just blindly believe that everything the complex biochemical food technology industry (whose primary motive is profit) puts into your foods is safe. Well, I have news for you.

It isn't safe. Over a long time it may have a very deleterious effect on your health and cause you to become susceptible to many degenerative conditions that slowly rob you of your quality of life.

A good example is the new controversy over glyphosate. Glyphosate is the active ingredient in weed killers. These chemicals are being sprayed on our crops to control weeds. Crops, such as soy, are being genetically modified (GMOs) to be resistant to glyphosate so only the weeds get killed. The World Health Organization has labeled glyphosate as "probably carcinogenic to humans." The inorganic materials in the herbicides are also causing concern. They are not tested as rigorously as the primary active ingredients. On testing, these chemicals were found to have crept into our food chain. Even some organically grown produce and breakfast foods have tested positive for glyphosate.

We all want to be active, energetic, mentally alert, and healthy when we grow older. We want to be able to enjoy the fruits of our labor. However, with the gradual poisoning of our bodies, that dream may not be obtainable.

Where is my proof? My proof is the number one and number two killers in the USA, Heart Disease and Cancer. They are not infectious diseases. They are diseases that are self-induced, either voluntarily or involuntarily, through deposits placed in our bodies by environmental exposure to processed foods and other pollutants. Other countries that do not eat the same types of foods we eat, do not have the same chronic diseases or cancers that we do.

However, they frequently develop our diseases when they start eating our food.

Remember, garbage in equals garbage out. If you put in too much garbage willingly, or unwillingly, you are going to have an immunologically frail body, rich in calories, poor in nutrients and loaded with toxins. We do not want to be like the falcons in Shenandoah National Park, slowly becoming extinct. Detoxification and cleaning your body out are the first secret to healthy aging.

CHAPTER 4

Caloric Restriction

When you observe people doing different things, such as walking, playing, moving from place to place, being involved in athletics, you'll notice a marked difference in activity and agility in significantly overweight people compared to thinner people:

What you actually see is less movement. There appears to be a geometrical proportion in increased weight to decreased mobility and decreased agility. How about coordination? How about shortness of breath with exertion?

What it boils down to is the greater your body fat, the less you are able to move swiftly and efficiently. You may say that is obvious. Yes it is, but how many times have you thought about it, and how many times have you thought about the consequences that this increased fat has on your entire life span?

If you are overweight, you have a significantly increased chance of developing a host of diseases from cardiovascular conditions to diabetes and arthritis. You also become a surgical risk candidate. Because of your increased fat your chances of complications are much greater, as are the chances of dying. Just think how hard it is to find a vein through all that fat? If movement is life, then less movement is less life and no movement is no life.

Do you want to truly live or do you want to barely live? That is the question you need to decide.

Why do I have a chapter on caloric restriction? Caloric restriction is so important in longevity that copping out of it would be a great disservice to you. Original studies on caloric restriction were conducted in 1935 by Dr. Clive McCay. He was able to extend the life of rats 50% by severely restricting their caloric intake. That's a whopping fifty percent! That's a lot.

I'm not talking about senile rats. I'm talking about active, vigorous, mentally alert rats. That research was largely ignored, although in the 1920s and 1930s outstanding research was performed on various topics that are pertinent and directly correlative to our health problems of today.

Let's get back to the general population and your observations. If you watch kids play on a playground, who does the most running, the heavy kids or the skinny kids? Who moves around more from place to place? Who is more agile? Who gives the appearance of vitality and youthfulness?

If you could take the heavy kids' movements and compare them to an older person's movements, you would find that the obese children have activity levels of older, less mobile people. Similarly, middle-aged, overweight people have the same activity level as extremely old people. I think you're starting to get the idea that the heavier you are, the less physical a life you will have. Your mind may be willing, but your body won't move.

I saw a patient today who was thin, muscular, and lean. I asked him if his grandparents were also thin; he said yes, they were. I asked how long they lived; he said, "Oh, they lived to be a hundred." I asked about his parents and he said, "Well, they're well into their late seventies and they're still in perfect health." Then, he added, "But we eat an Indian-type diet of fish and chicken."

I had another patient come in and I noticed that he was also in very good shape, and this man was well into his seventies. I said, "You seem to be in phenomenal shape." I asked, "How old was your father when he died?"

"Did I say my father was dead?" he replied. "My father is ninety-seven and he plays golf every day and goes dancing three times a week."

"That's remarkable. Well, how old was your grandfather when he died?"

"Did I say my grandfather died?" he answered. "My grandfather is a hundred and fifteen years old and just got married. Now he's expecting a child."

"That's really remarkable, somebody a hundred and fifteen years old wanting to get married and start a family."

"Did I say he wanted to get married?"

The purpose of the above stories, one true and the other made up, is that if you are calorically restricted and are relatively thin, you will have a much more vigorous, active, and potent lifestyle into old age.

The other day, I was driving by the Kids N' Kubs baseball field in downtown St. Petersburg, Florida. I had some time after lunch, so I decided to stop and watch these people play. They had a vigorous baseball game going on; good, solid hits to the outfield, line drives past the shortstop and second base, and decent runs to first base. There were even spectators in the bleachers watching.

I looked at every one of these players. They were almost all thin. A couple of them had slight potbellies, but nothing to be worried about. I talked to an elderly lady sitting next to the announcer and asked her about the team.

She said that "in order to qualify for the team, you have to be at least seventy-five years old, and those are the rookies." Her husband, who is the announcer, is eighty-eight. The president of the organization is ninety.

She pointed to a spry man walking quickly after picking up the bat from the batter. "He looks good and he runs good," she said. "He amazes me. And he's eighty-eight." I looked at the gentleman. He was thin and lean. He had the body language of a thirty-five-year-old. "A few have pot-bellies," the woman added. "They try to play, but they don't run as well."

Besides being active, the Kids N' Kubs are thin and they don't "act their age," they act young. As stated previously, movement is life. Consequently, the heavier you are, the less active you will be on a daily basis – this will lead to serious health issues in the long run.

What does the research show? I mentioned the original experiments from 1935, which were all but forgotten by modern medicine. This research was later resurrected in the early seventies by Dr. Roy Walford, a medical researcher from California.

Dr. Roy Walford was one of the participants and the medical person in the Biosphere II experiments near Tucson, Arizona. Biosphere II was a sealed, three-acre dome with its own ecosystems. Dr. Walford had noticed that, due to unanticipated restrictions of the food they were trying to grow in the Biosphere, participants were forced to cut diets down to 1800 calories per day.

He did repeated blood work on his fellow Biospherians and found that they were healthier with the reduced caloric diet. Since the participants had to grow their own food supply, they became more active and yet ate less. They lost weight and felt good. The changes he saw in them were similar to changes he observed in other calorically restricted species.

The diet that Clive M. McCay developed in 1935 at Cornell University was low in calories but high in nutrients. This high nutrient/low calorie diet enabled his rats, which were fed a severely caloric-restricted diet at near starvation levels, to live approximately 50% longer.

Since the early 1970s, Dr. Walford has been doing similar experiments on mice. In his mice experiments, a control group ate all they wanted, but the caloric restricted group had 40% fewer calories with all the nutrients they needed, including vitamins and minerals.

"What these mice have given mankind is perhaps the answer to a healthier, longer life," Dr. Walford stated. "They live a remarkable one-third longer than their well-fed counterparts. This is the first and only intervention proven to extend maximum life span throughout the animal kingdom."

According to Dr. Walford, "It works all the way across the animal kingdom, calorically restricted one-cell organisms, worms, mice, rodents, rats, fish, all live a great deal longer, equivalent to let's say 150 to 160 years in humans. So, it would be very surprising if it worked all across the animal kingdom, but not in humans."

Dr. Walford also backed up his statements by the research he had done in Biosphere II. He noted that the humans in the Biosphere II dome showed the same extensive physiological, biochemical, hormonal, and blood changes that rodents showed when they were calorically restricted.

In the Biosphere II experiment, Dr. Walford found that the men showed an average weight loss of 26 pounds and the women 15 pounds by eating 1800 calories. The blood pressure of the individuals fell sharply. Total cholesterol also dropped 35% on average. Dr. Walford also noted a large drop in white blood cell counts, which indicated strong immune systems. (Similar findings were seen in people doing intermittent fasting.)

Some of the primary indications of youth are agility, coordination, and activity level. Dr. Walford tested those indicators in a log-rolling contest for mice. The contest involved two mice balancing themselves on a log in water and trying to stay on. The less agile one fell off. Remember the game of two people balancing themselves on a log in water and trying to knock each other off? The one with the greater balance, agility, and dexterity was the winner. Do you think an older individual would be as agile in a log-rolling contest as a younger individual? One would generally expect the coordination and reflexes of the older one to be much slower and his balancing ability to also be greatly diminished, wouldn't you?

The same thing held true for the mice. When the caloric restricted mice were pegged against the mice that ate all they wanted, the calorically restricted mice were thinner, had shinier coats and were more aggressive and agile. These thin mice were able to stay on a rolling log much longer than the fully fed mice.

In other words, although they were the same chronological age, their biological ages were markedly different. They acted as if they were young.

The mice that ate as much as they wanted acted old and fell off the logs. Their reflexes were impaired. Their balance was impaired. Their coordination was impaired, and they lacked agility and endurance.

Now think about your experiences in observing people. Think about the people you have known who have been ill. Which ones show greater signs of youth, the overweight or the thin? How do they move? How are their reflexes? How quick are they? How fast do they walk?

The fewer calories you eat, the leaner you're going to be. As long as you eat a nutrient-rich diet, you're also going to be healthy, agile, mobile, and experience greater physical performance similar to that of your younger counterparts.

There was another experiment of interest done at the University of Wisconsin Primate Research Center where I studied. Dr. Rick Weindruch had been following Rhesus monkeys that were on a caloric-restricted (CR) diet. Since Rhesus monkeys live thirty to forty years, it was a longitudinal study.

The study began in 1989, and findings of this 20-year longitudinal study were published in *Science*, a research journal, in July 2009. The study stated that "In a population of Rhesus macaques maintained at the Wisconsin National Primate Research Center, moderate CR (caloric restriction) lowered the incidence of aging-related deaths. At the time point reported, 50% of control fed animals survived compared with 80% survival of CR animals. Further, CR delayed the onset of age-associated pathologies. Specifically, CR reduced the incidence of diabetes, cancer, cardiovascular disease, and brain atrophy. These data demonstrate that CR slows aging in a primate species." Remember, monkeys are the closest relatives to humans, as we are all primates.

After 20 years, 50% of the control animals were still alive – in that same time frame, 80% of caloric-restricted primates were still alive. That is a huge difference.

How would you like to improve your chances of not having diabetes, cancer, cardiovascular disease or brain atrophy?

If you slow down aging, you will have more time to enjoy life and to do the things you want to. After all, don't we want to be able to have as much fun as possible in our retirement? And to remember what we did in the past?

Jessie, a thin, spry, attractive, happy, 94 year old lady that I interviewed in Twillingate, Newfoundland, Canada stated "I do crossword puzzles all the time...it's good for the memory." "When your memory is gone, that's it, and you're gone." How true. I saw a large print book of crossword puzzles next to her rocker. She said that she didn't eat much, and got up out of her rocking chair to give me a copy of the exercises she did.

If you had compared the pictures of a typically caloric-restricted monkey and an unrestricted monkey who was able to eat what he wanted, similar to a typical American diet, you would have seen a huge difference in appearance. A typically unrestricted monkey looked old, had a very thin fur coat with bald patches, and a somewhat hunched back. The calorically restricted monkey had a youthful face, a lean body and a full, thick, fur coat. The difference in appearance between the caloric-unrestricted and restricted monkey was startling. It was like looking at a 40-year-old fit human, versus a 70-year-old unfit, sedentary, balding human.

In the first edition of this book, the data were not yet all in, yet changes were starting to appear. After 20 years, what a marked difference in appearance, health and longevity in the calorically restricted primates occurred. Just for curiosity, look at the pictures yourself on the internet. They were published in *Science*, on July 10, 2009. A picture is worth a thousand words.

By now I believe you're starting to understand how important caloric restriction is, as long as there are adequate nutrients.

The body only needs certain building blocks to function properly. When these requirements of trace minerals and vitamins are met, along with amino acids, and there is adequate bulk in our diet for motility of our gastrointestinal tract (enough volume to push through our gut so we can have a normal bowel movement), the body will work efficiently.

We will be much healthier than the individual who eats excessively and clogs up his cells with pesticides, hormones, heavy metals, unnatural fatty acids such as trans fatty acids, and thousands of other man-made chemicals that are hidden in our food chain.

Maintaining health is an ongoing process. It is a process which we have to continuously work at. If you want to live healthy into your old age and not be "old" when you're old, you need to plan ahead.

Nature has certain basic laws that need to be followed. There are no quick fixes, no operations, and no magic pills. What effort you put into your anti-aging program, you will receive back many times over when you reach eighty, ninety, or a hundred and more.

Dr. Walford was able to extend the life of his mice by a third in calorically restricting them to sixty percent of their normal caloric intake. The normal American diet consists of 2500 to 3500 calories, with some people eating considerably more than that.

If we apply the same ratios of caloric restrictions to our diets, we will be eating 1700 to 2000 calories per day. If we eat nutrient-rich, unprocessed, not chemically treated, pesticide-free foods, we should be able to get the same benefits as other animal species do by restricting the diet. That is, gaining a longer, healthier life span by at least a third. A one-third increase in our life span would allow us all to live between at least 100 and 120 years, some maybe even longer. I definitely feel that young, healthy, active, mentally alert 100-year-olds are going to be plentiful in this century if they follow the longevity programs as described in this book.

In the Wisconsin Primate Research Center study, each caloric-restricted animal's baseline food intake was reduced by 10 percent per month to reach a desired 30 percent reduction. This reduction would be about 1,750 to 2,450 calories per day for a typical person. It's a moderate reduction with proven health benefits in monkeys, our closest biological neighbors.

Remember, you reap what you sow. If you sow healthy seeds in a lean, chemically pure, fit body, you will reap a long, healthy, active, alert, joyful, fun life into a very young old age. There are the old-old and the young-old. You want to be in the young-old category.

So where do you start? A good place to start is to eat small meals throughout the day and not eat anything after supper. Another thing you could do is eat a big meal at lunchtime and a light meal in the evening, preferably consisting of either fruit or mixed vegetables with a little olive oil or canola oil and apple cider vinegar.

You could also have some protein consisting of beans, broiled cod or salmon, or free-range chickens (those whose feed has not had hormones or arsenic added). The important thing to remember is to eat early and keep your evening meal very light. It's best to eat your main meal during lunch if possible. Simply having an early supper and not eating afterwards is a good start toward caloric restrictions. If you eliminate supper all together, have a large lunch and a small snack at supper time, your body will love you.

We will go into nutrient recommendations further on in this book. You will have to figure out for yourself how to greatly reduce your caloric intake by eliminating fat foods, deep-fried foods, pastries and sweets and substituting nutrient-laden foods consisting of primarily pesticide-free fruits and vegetables.

Yes, you can occasionally splurge and treat yourself as long as you maintain a regular caloric-restricted diet of between 1750 to 2450 calories. Occasional palate alteration is not going to hurt you that much.

Talking about diabetes, in our teaching hospital we have an oncologist who slowly gained weight to the point where he developed hypertension and diabetes. What he decided to do surprised me. He went on an intermittent 5:2 fast, eating what he wanted for 5 days and 600 calories on his "fasting" days, and he lost 40 lbs. in 5 months. His hypertension went away as did his diabetes. He was so impressed with the results that he gave a grand rounds lecture for physicians to explain what could be achieved through intermittent fasting. He said it wasn't that hard, it's a goal like any other goal in life; you just don't eat, even if you are a little hungry, on your fasting days.

So plan ahead for a happy, active, joyful, alert retirement with a superb quality of life. Don't depend on that magic pill such as Rapamycin, an immune suppressant, or rely on having your blood transfused with young blood or plasma as a last ditch effort. Depend upon yourself now while you can. Stop eating junk. Reduce your calories drastically and you will reap the benefits at the later stages of your life, where it counts the most. You, too, can be like the eighty-eight year old baseball player who acts and behaves like he's thirty-five, full of energy and vitality, enjoying his life to the fullest.

CHAPTER 5

Physical Activity and Longevity

The most important secret of longevity is physical activity. Physical activity, along with caloric restrictions, requires the greatest amount of self-control and self-discipline. Since I am a specialist in rehabilitation, this is a topic dear to my heart. I have produced twenty-eight specific rehabilitative exercise videos (VCR exercises) to restore joint mobility and strengthen surrounding muscles.

I also provided lectures to international physicians interested in integrative medicine in the anti-aging course at the American College for Advancement of Medicine (ACAM). Most of these physicians did not fully realize the importance of physical activity in longevity. During my lecture, I asked everyone to stand in place and walk for the entire hour. I tried to maintain a fairly steady pace and I counted out the cadence for the doctors to walk in place. Periodically, during my lecture, I looked out at the audience to see how they were doing. I urged them to keep up the pace.

After fifteen minutes, and even after thirty minutes, a percentage of my audience stopped exercising or greatly slowed down. Yet, these were physicians interested in anti-aging. That was why they were taking the course. How can doctors, purporting to be pioneers in integrative medicine and preventative medicine, be in such poor shape? Have they merely substituted pill-pushing from big, mega-billion-dollar drug companies to vitamin-pushing, or were they truly serious in making a change in themselves and their patients?

I'm happy to say there were many in the audience who were vigorous in their exercise efforts, some even jumping up and down from one leg to the other, raising their knees high to get the full benefit of the exercise. Obviously there are some physicians who want to set good examples for their patients.

We live in a society of instant fixes. We want everything now. We want youth now. We want fun now. We want money now. We want things now on credit. We want self-gratification and self-indulgence now. Well, I hate to break the bad news to you, but it just does not work that way.

You can't cheat nature. The rules of nature have been laid down over millions of years. You must be physically active to maintain joint function, muscle tone, mental acuity, hormonal function, and crucial metabolic pathways, including blood sugar transfer from our blood to our cells. If you cheat nature, you cheat yourself.

Movement is life. Every atom in the universe has movement. Even steel atoms have movement. Cells have movement. Nerve and muscle cells have movement. A brain wave pattern involves movements. Our thoughts involve movements, with transfer of chemical messages from one cell to another. The basic law of motion is universal. Without movement, there is death.

One of the great baseball players of the twentieth century thought that life was like a bar of soap. You gradually wear it out until there is nothing left. In his time, it made sense.

As we've progressed into the 21st century, this view has shifted. We know much more about nerve transmission and mental acuity. We know you can take a feeble, frail, nursing home patient in his nineties and within two months, rehabilitate his muscle strength and increase it by 174%. We know that now. The baseball player didn't.

Muscular performance can be improved at any age. Muscle cells do not just wear away like a bar of soap. They can be rebuilt, re-toned, strengthened. Muscular strength and tone are directly related to your ability to be active when you are older. Why did the eighty-eight-year-old ball player at the Kids 'n Kubs baseball field walk with a brisk pace, pick up a bat, and walk back to the dugout just like a forty year old? Because he maintained his muscle tone and activity level. He was continuously active when he got older. In other words, he put in effort.

You have got to plan ahead. What you put in is exactly what you get out. There are no shortcuts. I know how hard it is to get out there and exercise three times a week. But I'll help you. At the end of this chapter, I'll give you the Lenhart Physical Activity Formula for Anti-Aging, derived after considerable research and analysis of hundreds of research articles, as well as personal experience through observation of patients and neighbors.

Sixty percent of the U.S. population is overweight or obese. An even greater percentage is inactive. Let's look at those statistics in economic terms. How many hundreds of billions of dollars have been made by the fast food industry to put on those wasted pounds? How many more billions were made by the biochemical industry to invent and process food so that it stays fresh forever, looks good, and tastes good? These chemists make a lot of money inventing chemicals to artificially fertilize the soil and kill all the pests in it, chemicals to grow food rapidly, create pest resistant plants and produce chemicals to preserve food and maintain its texture. They also genetically modified our food. As a matter of fact, they are engineering pesticides to be built into the plants so spraying of crops will not be necessary. Soon they will produce genetically altered beef and chickens.
Livestock will grow faster and slaughterhouses will become more profitable.

Let's continue the economic aspect of your behavior further. Due to poor lifestyle habits, the medical industry will get larger and larger. Baby boomers grew up on fast food, additives, chemicals, comfortable couches, easy chairs, high fat and high-sugar munchies. As they age, drug companies and some hospitals will make lots of money because those Boomers will need continual medical care.

Drug companies will compete at breakneck speed to create new magic pills to fight these diseases we have due to our poor lifestyles. The government will be near bankruptcy because of the high costs of Medicare and Medicaid to supply all the services to those who didn't take care of their bodies and minds and didn't plan ahead.

Baby boomers are retiring at the rate of ten thousand a day. That is a huge stressor on our health care system and something has to give. Less coverage? More co-pay? Use your imagination as to how the government will react to this extra burden on the system.

If you don't use it, you lose it.

If you sit back, relax, and do not put any effort into a preventive anti-aging health care program, you will suffer the consequences in the later stages of life.

Increased physical activity is absolutely the cheapest, most efficient, most effective way to increase your chances of prolonging your life substantially, and at the same time, decrease all the diseases that plague us in our older age. Physical activity done on a consistent, regular basis is, just by itself, the best healthy aging treatment available, even without adding all the other possibilities mentioned in this book. The more of the Longevity Secrets you undertake, however, the greater you increase your odds for a healthier, disease-free, mentally alert retirement.

About thirty years ago, I moved into a neighborhood in which my neighbor was a very elderly gentleman; at least, he looked elderly. He was seventy-three-years-old, frail, pale, and walked really slowly. I saw him start to go on short walks up and down the block on a daily basis. Eventually, he started biking and increased his distance progressively.

Over the years, as I watched this gentleman, I saw this old, frail person turn into a vigorous, strong, youthful individual. By the time he was eighty-five, he was walking at about a 3.5 mph (5.8 km/hr) pace in the morning and evening. If you saw him from the rear, not knowing how old he was, you would swear that he walked and looked like a forty-year-old. His legs had good muscle tone. He had a spring to his walk. He walked deliberately with a cadence and arm swing that one sees in younger people.

Before this gentleman started his walking program, he was very, very ill and near death. The persistent, continuous physical activity that he did not only helped him to recover, but also to grow biologically younger. It increased his stamina and kept him from developing many age-related diseases.

One day, I asked him what else he did to keep himself so young and fit, and he said he lifted weights on a regular basis to keep up his muscle tone.

I have since observed other individuals following a similar protocol of continued physical activity who were able to stay young well into their eighties and nineties.

Dancing is another excellent means of maintaining physical activity into old age. I noticed this with my uncle, who went ballroom dancing twice a week. He died in his nineties. He did not even follow any other longevity programs, as outlined in this book. All he did was increase his physical activity by dancing well into old age.

Through my ballroom and swing dance experiences, I have been able to observe very healthy retirees who are my dance partners. Some of those ladies are proud to tell me that they are 85 or 87 years old and that dancing keeps them going. After several years of observing how alert and fit these dancers were, I decided to write *Dance to Live*. The book spells out all of the health, longevity and social benefits of dancing. You will be surprised what dancing does for your balance, muscle strength, bones, endurance, social interaction, coordination, and mind.

Why is maintaining physical activity so important? It preserves and strengthens your muscles, joints, ligaments, tendons, and bones. At the same time, it conditions your cardiovascular system and increases waste elimination, which ties into "Detoxification", the third chapter of this book. By pumping your muscles, you are forcing excretion of waste products that have accumulated. As well, increased cardiovascular stress from exercise conditions and strengthens your heart.

You may be asking at this time, "What does exercise have to do with conditioning my bones?" To tell you the truth, most doctors don't know either. Only those physicians who have studied radiology realize that there is a direct correlation of both growth and strength, which is directly proportional to the stress placed on the bone.

There is a law in radiology and bone growth called the Wolff's Law, stating that the bone will directly remodel itself based upon the force applied to it. In other words, putting it in laymen's terminology, the bone gets stronger only if it is stressed. If you do not put stress on the bone, it becomes soft, weak, brittle, and subject to breaks.

What is one of the most common disabilities that occurs in older individuals? Hip fractures and other bone fractures. When people age, they don't stress their bones enough to maintain their strength. Any type of small trauma can cause bones to break. When bones break, people become immobilized. Then begins a downward cycle.

Immobility leads to muscle wasting. Muscle wasting leads to incapacitation. Incapacitation leads to further degeneration, loss of the ability to perform activities of daily living, and eventually, death.

How many elderly people have you known who broke a major bone, such as a hip, never recovered, and rapidly thereafter, ended up dying?

Did you know that one week of bed rest causes you to lose twenty percent of your muscle mass? Every subsequent week of bed rest causes you to lose another twenty percent of the residual muscle mass. It does not take a genius to figure out how weak you can become, in a very short period of time, by not moving or stressing your muscles.

If you don't believe me, look at the astronauts. What happens after they return from space missions? Do they have to be helped out of their space vehicles? We've seen it many times. They come out frail, weak, and unsteady on their feet. That's because they didn't have the opportunity to stress their bones and muscles adequately in space.

It all goes back to the same rule. If you don't use it, you lose it ... rapidly.

Let's get back to the bed rest patients. How long do you think it would take for them to regain their muscle strength if they lose twenty percent of their muscle mass with one week of bed rest? In order to regain that, it would require maximum contraction of the muscles, on a daily basis for one week, to regain only ten percent of the muscle mass they have lost. Now, they have to do this for every muscle group that has been weakened. That's a heck of a lot of work to regain ten percent.

It doesn't seem fair, does it, but that's the way biology works. You must continue to use your muscles, ligaments, and tendons, and also put stress on your bones, to maintain function and prevent disability.

If you look at the Kids 'n Kubs 1998 world champion baseball team in St. Petersburg, whose members were all over eighty, you will see that they have maintained a joyful, physical-activity-filled retirement. They have continuously moved their bodies, stressed their joints, ligaments, and tendons and constantly maintained muscle tone, which preserved their joints, bones, and overall health.

Going back to my rehabilitation literature--let's go over what happens to your body through inactivity. Let's see how many diseases you will recognize simply due to immobility. By my explaining the body's responses to immobility, you will be able to understand the beneficial effect of physical activity almost immediately, as immobility and inactivity mimic the effects of aging.

Your central nervous system, which is the electrical system of your body, reacts to immobilization by decreasing your sensations. It decreases your ability to move. Your motions change, as well as your behavior, and you start to lose intellectual ability. In other words, you cannot think as clearly.

Your muscular system makes all your bones move and gives you propulsion. It allows you to stand, breathe, sit, and walk. Not only does it lose up to twenty percent of its initial strength during one week of bed rest, but with immobilization, the endurance decreases, the muscles atrophy, and you lose coordination.

What about your bones? Previously, I mentioned that bones react to the stresses placed upon them. With extended immobilization you get osteoporosis. You've heard of that, I'm sure. Osteoporosis is the thinning of the bones. This thinning leads to fractures, disability, and eventually early death.

You can also get fibrosis. This means scar tissue forms at your joints causing them to eventually fuse so that you cannot move. Well, that's a bummer. If you can't move, you're in a dying state because the reverse of dying is movement.

Then there's your cardiovascular system, your heart and circulation. Immobility leads to decreased heart rate resulting in low blood pressure and, when you stand up or sit up, it may cause you to pass out. You may also get blood clots. Blood clots lead to the inability to breathe and suffocation, or, if they go to the brain, stroke.

It all happens because you are not moving. You can also get what is called a decreased cardiac reserve. The heart just cannot pump well enough to get the blood to the vital organs and muscles.

What about your breathing? What happens to your breathing if you get immobilized? Well, you can't breathe as well. You cannot take in as much air due to what is known as a restrictive impairment. You're not getting as much oxygen because there is less oxygen going across your lung membranes, and you need that oxygen to live. One of the worst things that can happen is that you can't cough as much. So, what's the big deal?

Well, just think about it. We have to cough to get "crud" out of our lungs. If we accidentally aspirate something, have a cold or mucous builds up in our lungs, we have to be able to cough and move it out. If you cannot cough, you'll get a major infection because the lungs will fill up with fluid. That increased fluid is a great opportunity for bacteria to set in, producing fever and pneumonia. If a virus gets in, you get viral pneumonia which we cannot treat with antibiotics. Pneumonia can lead to death. Unless you have great resistance, which you don't because you have been immobilized, you will most likely meet your maker. All of this because you are not moving, which is something that is preventable, for the most part. Unfortunately, it's a downward spiral.

How about your digestive system? You lose your appetite and become constipated. What about your kidneys? You end up peeing more. You may end up losing some of your sodium, which is very important for your body. You could end up losing calcium. That would explain why you become osteoporotic; calcium is taken out of your bones. You might end up getting kidney stones, which are extremely painful.

What about your skin? The skin starts to atrophy. Atrophy is a wearing away, or thinning of, the skin and you could end up getting bed sores. Bed sores can lead to big ulcers, which lead to infections. Not a pretty sight.

What I have described to you is how the systems in the body break down just by immobilization and inactivity. If you look at older, frail, immobile individuals, you will see the same symptoms I described. It is a cascade of events. One thing leads to another, and another, until eventually death occurs.

Let me give you an example about the oldest man in Japan. He lived in Okinawa, one of the blue zones in the world where people live for a long time. It is an island noted for its high nutrient foods, low-calorie, restricted diets. He reached 112 years of age. He did agricultural work until he was eighty-five. That means he was doing hard, physical labor to keep his muscles and joints moving.

He remained active after he stopped doing farm work. He was a Type A personality, very active mentally and physically. His blood tests were normal. He was able to take care of himself completely until he was 108 years old. When something happened to him, and he had to go to a hospital, well, guess what happened?

Once he got to the hospital, he lost control of his life, individuality and movements. What happens in a hospital? Immobilization. He deteriorated rapidly. His sharp mind slipped into dementia within 3 years. This is a good example of what immobility does to you in rapid progression, especially if you are older.

What about immobility of the brain? The Use It or Lose It principle holds true in all the systems of our body. Your ability to think clearly and make decisions rapidly is based upon the number of dendrites (connections) you have in your brain. Dendrites are like small branches in an oak tree that fan out and give the tree its shape. Those branches talk to each other.

Let's assume your mind is a forest, with intermingling branches, and the trees are tightly packed together. The more branches you have, the closer together the trees become.

Now, assume that there is a small monkey jumping from one branch to another, and a leopard is chasing him. The more these little branches are intertwined between the trees, the faster he'll be able to run away, making unimpeded connections from one tree to the next, and eluding his predator.

There was a study done on rats placed into a playpen for an hour a day where they were given objects that varied daily. With some free space, these rats had the freedom to explore new environments. It was a physically charged and very intellectually stimulating experience because the rats had to crawl up and down and around all these objects.

Another group of rats didn't get the exercise and were not put into this mentally challenging environment. At the end of the experiment, the rats were sacrificed and their brains studied. Guess what they found?

The brains that were physically and mentally challenged had a large number of connectors (dendrites), like the sprouting branches of trees. Coincidentally, these dendrites are evident in very young people because they are still learning a lot of new things, creating new connections. The rats not physically and mentally stimulated had considerably fewer connectors, or fewer branches to make connections. That's similar to older people who are not mentally challenged.

You see, people used to think, just like the old bar of soap I mentioned before, that generally, your brain just wears out, deteriorates, and shrinks in size. If you take MRIs of people's brains, you will see atrophy in older individuals. There is a lot more fluid and a lot less gray matter, which is the stuff that does the thinking. However, it does not have to be that way.

There is a group of researchers studying nuns in Mankato, Minnesota. They live in a convent and routinely live past their nineties. These nuns were progressive educators, so they donated their brains to science after they died, a noble cause.

It was discovered that the college-educated ones lived longer, and because the religious order believed that an idle mind is the devil's playground, the nuns constantly did brain exercises and crossword puzzles, played Jeopardy on television, and performed other activities that constantly stimulated their minds. On autopsy, they found the nuns all had extensive brain dendrite formation at the time of death due to the intellectual stimulation. In other words, they were mentally young. The researchers noted that the ones who stayed mentally active did not suffer from dementia as much as those who didn't.

Newer research is also finding that people who have lost some of their intellectual capacity can regain it by constantly stimulating their brains. They can actually grow new dendrites, not just keep the ones they have, which is a very, very encouraging finding. You can grow intellectually younger just by stressing your brain and making it work, constantly teaching it new things. It is that same Use It or Lose It philosophy.

The more I started thinking about this, the more I started thinking about my own life, how I am constantly changing and learning new things. There must be some kind of hidden signal telling me that it is time for me to become intellectually challenged again. Once I have learned one topic and used it for a while, I tend to move on to another field of medicine, or business, or computer science that stimulates my intellect. I go to grand rounds weekly to learn about new advances in medicine. Grand rounds are lectures given in a teaching hospital to further educate physicians and resident physicians. In St Petersburg, Florida, we have two top notch resident teaching hospitals, Bayfront Medical Center and Johns Hopkins All Children's Hospital, that provide me continuous medical education. I also like working on several things at the same time with different intellectually stimulating capacities. Every different thing you do stimulates a different part of your brain.

Let's go back to the Darwinian theory of evolution. Darwin was the guy that did much of his research in the Galapagos Islands, off the coast of Ecuador, where he discovered that different birds developed in different ways, became highly specialized in food gathering, and had high survival rates. He had a group of finches that were divergent; they could eat different types of seed and survive in different environments. Other finches could eat only one type of seed. If that plant became extinct, that species also became extinct.

Your brain works in the same way. It has to have a large variety of stimuli to keep it going and keep it growing. If you develop only one specific aspect of your brain, the other aspects tend to wither away because they're not being used and not being stimulated.

You become one-sided and, as your spouse may think, boring. I hate to say this, but people who only talk about one thing, know one thing, or work at one thing are not as interesting as people who are educated about several topics and can hold a variety of intellectual conversations. A quest for knowledge is one of the most enduring qualities a human can have. That is what differentiates him or her from other mammalian creatures such as apes.

Let's summarize this subject by reminding you that the more connectors you have, the better your ability to make connections. It holds true in the business world just as much as in your brain. The second part is that intellectual stimulation can cause dendrites to branch out, creating networks of new connections producing neuroplasticity.

Muscles. What do muscles do? It seems obvious. They hold up your skeleton, protect your organs, and provide movement to the bony part. They must be used constantly to maintain performance and keep you alive. If you don't believe me, look at people suffering from muscular dystrophy. You've seen the telethons on television about muscular dystrophy, but you have probably never fully realized what that disease does. It slowly destroys your muscles until they wear out. When the muscles wear out, you can't even sit in a wheelchair. After a while you can't breathe. That is how important your muscles are. Your heart is a big muscle.

Bones. Bones provide a framework, something to attach things to and provide structure, like your house foundation and outside walls.

They hold things up. They are attachment points for muscles. They facilitate movements through joints. Bones allow the joints to move in and out or in circles, as different joints in your body do, including talking, as I'm doing right now dictating this book. However, in order for those bones to work properly and not break and fall apart, they need stress to maintain their mineral content and give them strength.

Bones have an internal honeycomb structure (trabeculae) which, like the Eiffel tower, use grid work to give them strength. If your bones are not constantly stressed and moved, they will lose that grid work.

When you lose some of that grid work, what happens to the structure? It weakens. Just think, if you took half the supporting structures out of the Eiffel Tower and a big wind came along, do you think the Tower would stay standing or do you think it would collapse? The same thing happens to your bones. Bones have to be stressed to stay healthy.

Bone is constantly reinforcing itself by any stress put on it to make sure it is strong enough to bear weight. So, overweight people gradually get stronger bones because they have more weight to carry. However, there is a down side to it: the bone joints cannot bear the weight as easily so they wear out.

Bone joints are made of cartilage and cartilage does not rebuild itself as easily as bones do to accommodate the stress placed upon it. Large people develop bad knees and bad joints because too much stress is placed upon those joints. However, if these joints are used constantly and lubricated through motion, there is less chance of them wearing out and a greater chance of new layers of cartilage forming over the joint.

There was a study done of a one-year walking program for women. What they found was that over one year of walking, those women had an increase of calcium in the top of the hip joint. However, there was no increase of calcium inside the wrist bones. Since women, in general, are prone to hip fractures, it showed that walking increased the strength of their hips. However, because the stress was only placed upon the hip joints and not the wrists joints, the extra bone deposits were placed where the stress was placed, in the hips.

So, what are the benefits of healthy bones, muscles, and ligaments? You get movement without impediment or disease. You get movement without pain. Isn't that wonderful? You prevent bone damage. You prevent muscular or ligament destruction. You gain power, speed, mobility, freedom, and a greater quality of life. You prevent debilitation and death. Use It or Lose It.

You may be saying, "That's fine, but I'm ninety. I didn't know about all that data. I didn't read this book till now." I have good news for you. A group of ninety-year-olds, sitting around in a nursing home with nothing to do, agreed to participate in a strengthening program. They did eight weeks of high intensity resistance training. The age group was eighty-seven to ninety-six. They trained one muscle group, the quadriceps, which is in the front of your thigh. In just eight weeks, they found increased strength of 174%. By strengthening that one muscle group their walking speed increased by 48%. These were eighty-seven to ninety six year-olds! They were able to rebuild their muscle mass and regain strength by 174%. To me, that is remarkable. It tells me that Use It or Lose It does not necessarily mean lose it forever. You can regain it at any age. Remember, movement is life.

Take a look at John Glenn, a seventy-seven-year-old astronaut. That's right, at seventy-seven-years-old, he returned to space. NASA scientists said he handled the rigors of space every bit as well as astronauts half his age. He suffered no more bone-mass loss or muscle loss than any of the younger astronauts. His heart rate before, during, and after the flight was actually better than the average of twelve, younger, male astronauts. Isn't that amazing? The message is clear. At seventy-seven you can do as well as a forty-year-old astronaut.

Glenn walked several miles a day, which I believe is the main reason he did so well. He also did some weight training and ate a balanced diet. Dr. David Williams, director of NASA's Life Science

Division and a former shuttle astronaut himself, stated that Glenn challenged the widespread notion that all seniors are frail individuals.

John Glenn did just as well as his younger counterparts. He spent four nights in a wired-up sleep suit. He provided seventeen blood samples and wore a small data recorder for twenty-four hours to monitor his heart rate. He also swallowed a capsule holding a radio transmitter and temperature sensor. How much more evidence do you need to see that at just about any age you can become young again through physical activity? Glenn conditioned himself to the level of a young person. If he had previously lost any functions, he regained them.

An interesting finding was that, like all other astronauts, Glenn experienced some balance problems once he returned to earth, but he recovered just as quickly as the other astronauts, which surprised the scientists. Many elderly people have difficulty with balance. A study that measured the effects of physical activity and calcium intake on the bone mass of healthy women of different ages found that, when taken alone, calcium had no effect on their bone mineral density. However, the people who exercised had a five percent increase in the bone mineral density in the exercised bones. Remember, I mentioned that you have to put stress on the bone in order for it to grow. However, there was no increase in bone mineral density in the nonweight-bearing bones that were not exercised.

The older you are, the more benefits your bones have from exercise. Exercise of weight bearing bones builds mineral content, size, and strength.

Another important component of physical activity is that exercise decreases diabetes and reduces the risk of non-insulin-dependent diabetes. There are a number of studies showing the benefits of exercise on reducing the risk of diabetes.

Diabetes naturally raises one's blood sugar levels. Normally there is a decline in insulin sensitivity associated with aging, inactivity, and obesity. If you lose weight, as the previous chapter discussed, and increase your physical activity, you will increase your insulin sensitivity and decrease your risk of diabetes. Diabetes is a chronic condition that greatly accelerates aging and often leads to premature death.

There was a study done in Finland of 898 men. The men were subjected to moderately intense physical activity at high levels of cardio-respiratory fitness. It was found that after four years, the more active individuals had a reduced risk of non-insulin-dependent diabetes mellitus by forty-four percent. That is very significant-- physical activity reduces your chance of diabetes by almost half. If you lose weight, you will do even better.

They also took the overweight, high blood pressure people in this group, who had a positive family history of diabetes and who were engaged in moderate to intense physical activity at least forty minutes a week, and reduced their risk of non-insulin dependent diabetes by fifty-four percent, compared to those who did not participate in such activities. What this is telling you is that the fatter you are, the more out of shape you are, and the more risk you have, the greater you will benefit from exercise. It is never too late to start a physically active program.

Another interesting thing that happens when you become physically active is that you increase your growth hormone level. There was another study that measured the hormone, mineral and cardiovascular levels of endurance-trained postmenopausal women and sedentary women.

The endurance-trained postmenopausal women (most likely greater than forty-five to fifty years of age) had lower body fat, lower weight, and higher aerobic capacity. When normalized for weight, the bone mineral density was higher in the spine. The interesting point was that the growth hormone level had increased.

Growth hormone is something I will talk about in a later chapter. It has been associated with youth. The theory is, the greater your growth hormone level, the more youthful characteristics you will have, such as a leaner body mass (less fat), more endurance, and a younger appearance. Exercise naturally increases your growth hormone level.

You might say, "Well, that's fine, but I've abused my body all these years. This isn't going to do me any good now." You are wrong!

The more you abused your body in the past, the greater your benefits. It has been proven over and over again, in numerous studies, that people in terrible shape can benefit greatly from physical activity. As a matter of fact, they have the most to gain. because they are the closest to the grave.

Some of the major impact studies I consider to be significant were done at Harvard University (the Harvard Alumni Health Study), at the Cooper Clinic in Dallas, Texas (a very well-known aerobic and cardiovascular clinic), in Hawaii (The Honolulu Heart Program), and in Finland, where they studied twins.

In the Harvard study, they took 17,321 men and studied them for approximately twenty-five years. They concluded that the men who were vigorously active had about fifteen to twenty-five percent lower chance of dying. Physical activity also decreased coronary artery disease, decreased high blood pressure, decreased non-insulin-dependent diabetes, decreased colon cancer, and increased life. One of the findings was that only vigorous activity had the remarkable difference of prolonging life. One had to expend about 1500 calories a week. Of the 17,321 men studied, there were 259 deaths of the vigorously active individuals and 380 deaths among the non-vigorously active individuals. That's a big difference. There was a direct relationship between total physical activity and mortality. What does that mean?

That means, the more active they were, to a certain limit, the less chance there was of them dying. Of the less active men, there were 121 more deaths. That is, almost one-third more deaths occurred because they were physically inactive.

At the Cooper Clinic in Dallas, Texas, researchers wanted to know if people who were initially in very poor condition could benefit from physical activity. They studied 9,777 men, ages 22 to 80, with a five-year follow-up. They found, as expected, people who were fit at the beginning and end of the study had the lowest death rate. However, the people who were unfit, and became fit during the five-year follow-up study, had a forty four percent reduction in the risk of death. This included all causes of death.

This should hit you between the eyes like a sledge hammer. If you can decrease your chance of dying by forty-four percent, or almost half, for all causes of death, wouldn't you jump at it?
How much more proof do you need to get off your butt and get going? Are you going to spend all your money when you get older on doctors, hospitals, and nursing homes? It is your choice.

Remember, exercise pumps out toxins. It prolongs life. Even walking is more fun if you go with a friend or family member, and it's a great time for bonding. Let's focus on walking. The Honolulu Heart Program study of retired men took 707 non-smokers, aged 61 to 81, and did a twelve-year follow-up. They recorded the distance these people walked. What they found was that the more miles a person walked per day, the lower the probability of dying.

The men who walked less than one mile a day died twice as fast as those that walked two miles a day. Their death rate was 40.5% versus 23.8% for those who walked two miles a day. What does that tell you?

Based upon this study, and other studies I have reviewed and lectured on, the magic number is two miles a day or more. Guess what else they found?

The most common cause of death in the 61 to 81 year old age group was cancer. The death rate of the people who died of cancer alone, and who walked less than one mile a day, was 13.4%. Among those who walked more than two miles a day, the death rate from cancer was 5.3%. That means those who walked less than one mile a day had twice the chance of dying from cancer than those who walked two miles, or more, per day. What a difference just one mile makes. Isn't that amazing?

That extra mile must trigger very important protective mechanisms in the body that keep your chemistry in balance, keep your body from going haywire, pumping out the toxins, increasing your cardiovascular fitness, as well as increasing the oxygenation and nutrition to your cells.

Whenever I have a chance to learn from my patients about aging and longevity, I jump at the chance. Recently, I had a hair stylist who came in as a patient. I found out that she worked in several adult-living facilities, which I thought was quite a niche market for a beautician. I quizzed her about her observations of her older clients, questions primarily dealing with their health, alertness, and what kind of clients they were.

One interesting observation she spoke of was that the hundred-year-olds she does hair for are more active, walk better, and have a much better attitude about life than the seventy-five to eighty-year-olds. She also said that their minds and memories are better.

Another point was that the hundred-year-olds were more resilient. They could overcome setbacks better and were much more pleasant to deal with than the sickly seventy-five to eighty-year-olds.

She said that the younger ones who were sickly, less active, and not as alert mentally always worried about things. They talked about negative things all the time, worrying that they'd break their hip someday. The ones who were sick always talked about being sick. The optimistic patients, however, never seemed to get as ill. The older patients seemed to live for the moment. They enjoyed life and they overcame obstacles through a positive mental attitude and an active lifestyle.

Those were interesting comments because they mirrored exactly what I have been finding in my own research and observations. The more active you are, the less time you have to worry. The less you worry, the fewer chances you will have of developing a physical ailment that can greatly debilitate you and lead you to an earlier grave. There is no reason to constantly worry about your physical state because you can do something about it.

There was another study done at the Cooper Clinic in Dallas, this one involving 25,000 men and 7,000 women. Researchers wanted to determine how people benefited from physical activity regardless of the shape they were in when they started. The study lasted nineteen years. Low, moderate, and high fitness levels were established for smokers, people with high cholesterol, high blood pressure, and other health conditions.

They found: 1. That low fitness was an important precursor to mortality, meaning the less fit you were, the greater your chance of getting ill; and 2. That the protective effect of fitness held for smokers as well as nonsmokers, for those with and without elevated cholesterol, and for unhealthy and healthy persons.

Everyone benefited from increased physical activity. People with low cardio-respiratory fitness benefited, as did those with moderate and high cardio-respiratory fitness, and as differentiated by smokers and nonsmokers.

Every category improved with fitness. Those with normal, moderate and high blood pressure all systematically improved after an exercise program. The same thing was true for people who were frequently ill.

Remember the neighbor I mentioned at the beginning of this chapter, and how I first met him when he was in his seventies? When I moved out of the neighborhood, he was well into his eighties and was in better shape than he'd been in his early seventies. That same observation I had of this one subject was observed at the Cooper Clinic with 32,000 subjects, and which was also the same observation my hair stylist patient noticed in her adult-living facility centenarians.

By the way, did you know that exercise also decreases breast cancer by 20 to 33 percent? There were a couple of studies done, about three years apart, in Norway and in the United States, which came up with these conclusions.

No matter what you say, some people will always be skeptical because they don't want to put in the effort. They think they are doomed. They think it is in their genes. They say, "Whatever happens, happens. I was destined to have cardiovascular disease, or cancer, or diabetes. . . ." They just give up.

I knew there would be objections to my findings, so I dug deeper into the literature and found a study done in Finland, which was titled, "Relationship of Leisure Time, Physical Activity, and Mortality, The Finnish Twin Cohort Study." They knew that physical activity and fitness were believed to reduce premature mortality. What they did not know was whether genetic factors modified this effect (the 'It's in your genes' hypotheses). They went on to study twins. Twins have the same parents, the same environment, the same food. Identical twins have the exact same genes because they come from the same egg.

In this Finnish twin cohort study, done between 1977 and 1994, they took 7,925 healthy men and 7,977 healthy women from ages 25 to 64, and they classified them into conditioning exercisers and sedentary people. The conditioning exercisers walked vigorously for thirty minutes at least six times a month. The other group had no leisure physical activity. (I consider thirty minutes six times per month to be almost nothing. However, they considered that conditioning.) Even with that minimal effort, the study results of the twins, in which one died during the studied period, showed the odds for death was 66 percent for occasional exercisers and 44 percent for conditioning exercisers.

That means that the people who walked vigorously at least thirty minutes for at least six times a month had a 21 percent lower chance of dying than the occasional exercisers;.

When all the results from all the twins were compared and adjusted for age and sex, you had a 71 percent chance of dying as often as a sedentary exerciser if you were an occasional exerciser, and a 57 percent chance of dying as often as a sedentary person if you were a conditioning exerciser. You had a 29 percent less chance of dying if you exercised occasionally and 43 percent less chance of dying if you exercised vigorously. To me, those are remarkable figures.

Based upon the twins studied, if you exercise vigorously only six times a month for thirty minutes by walking, you reduce your death rate chance by more than 40 percent. The overall conclusion of this study was that familial factors did not explain the mortality differences by physical activity found in an individual-based analysis. Occasional and conditioning twin exercisers had reduced their risk of death significantly compared to sedentary twins.

You should re-read that last line several times until it sinks in. One interesting finding in this study, when I reviewed the raw data, was that women seemed to do better than the men. If you took the sedentary women and assumed that they had a 100% chance of dying at the end of the study, the conditioning women had a 24% chance of dying. That means they reduced their chance of death by 76% just by walking vigorously thirty or more minutes six times a month. It's amazing. Absolutely amazing.

So wake up. The only thing that is keeping you from increasing your life span is you.

There have been other studies done that measure the benefits of lifestyle activity during the day. As expected, people who were more physically active during the day had better blood pressure and lower body fat. What they are showing you is that it is not always necessary to have a structured physical activity program to get beneficial results from physical activity. However, the people in that group alone, who did have a structured program, had greater improvement in their cardio-respiratory fitness than those who were just more physically active in the daytime. So, you will get more benefit out of a structured program than you do on an irregular basis.

Movement is life.

If you don't move, you die. It is as simple as that.

You get progressive decompensation if you don't move due to lack of muscle and joint stress, which can lead to rapid death.

These statements above are extremely important because they wrap up, in a nutshell, exactly what happens to you if you are not physically active. If you do not have good muscle strength and coordination, you will trip and fall more frequently and will not recover as easily.

If your bones are weak because they have not been stressed, you break them more often, which will lead to further disability and bed rest, which can lead to pneumonia and eventual death, or you may have a greater chance of developing colon cancer, heart disease, and as shown in the Honolulu study, a fifty percent greater chance of developing cancer just by not being physically active.

Did you know that falling is the number one cause of injury in people 65 years old or older? Also, that the risk of death three months after a hip fracture is five to eight times higher? One in three adults age 65 and older falls each year and the cost to the US health system in 2010 for those falls was $30 billion. A walking program, as described in this book, could greatly reduce those falls and a dancing program reduce it even further.

The World Health Organization (WHO) stated in 2015 that "Levels of physical activity are decreasing and sedentary behaviors increasing with detrimental consequences." They also included cardiovascular disease, diabetes, hyperglycemia, hypertension and cancer, along with obesity.

There has been some concern in the literature about over exercising, but in 2011, in the *Journal of Sports Medicine*, a report about cyclists addressed this subject. The title was "Increased Average Longevity among the Tour de France Cyclists" who did the grueling race between 1930 and 1964. Guess what they found? Half the general population in that region of Europe died at 73.5 years-of-age whereas the Tour de France participants died at 81.5 years. The extreme athletes lived 8 years longer. I found similar data with Copenhagen joggers and Polish Olympic athletes. In the *American Journal of Epidemiology*, June 2012, a research article titled "Longevity in Male and Female Joggers: The Copenhagen City Heart Study," found that "Jogging was associated with significantly lower all-cause mortality." All-cause mortality means fewer deaths from all illnesses. Now that's a big deal.

Posture

I decided to include posture in this edition because many people are not aware of the importance it has in our longevity program.

Why is posture important? It is important because it affects how our body ages and the health problems we may have because of poor posture. We need to hold ourselves as erect as possible with our head straight, our shoulders back and our bellies tucked in.

Poor sitting and lying habits can affect our spine which can lead to deformities, degeneration and arthritis.

When you select a chair, sofa or recliner, make sure that the area you sit on from front to back is approximately the same length as the back of your knees to your back. You should sit with your back supported. I had a doctor friend that purchased northern European furniture because it looked modern and "cool." The problem was that the seat area was much too wide and he had to slouch a lot to lean against the back. He was trained in intensive care medicine and had no idea that he was ruining his spine and health by the sofa he was sitting on at home while watching television or reading.

When you are constantly slouched, the ligaments in the front of your spine become contracted. Contracted ligaments cause your spine to bow out in back like a humpback. This contraction leads to poor walking posture with your head leaning forward and down. The slouching can also permanently deform your spine, cause arthritis and decrease your lung cavity so that you cannot breathe in as much air. You need to oxygenate you tissues as much as possible when you are exercising. If there is less room for your lungs to expand you cannot breathe in as much air. There is a lot of research done in this field but unfortunately most doctors, unless trained in rehab, chiropractic, or pulmonary medicine, don't know anything about it. Too many pillows can also cause your neck and upper back to be deformed. Cell phones are creating another problem. People are constantly looking down trying to read their text messages. This continued neck flexion may affect your normal spinal curves and cause lasting deleterious effects. Posture is important and we need to pay attention to it.

"Okay, okay. I've had enough data. Now tell me what to do." Here it is.

What are your exercise options? There are different types of exercise: 1) Cardiovascular/aerobic exercise such as running, bicycling, speed walking, elliptical machines, stair climbing 2) Strength building or bulking exercise like resistance training or weightlifting with free weights and machines 3) Load-bearing such as walking, roller blading, skiing, jumping or running. Load-bearing strengthens bones. 4) Rowing, which combines many different types of movements; it allows cardiovascular and abdominal muscle strength building 5) Range of motion exercises such as swimming, jumping jacks, stretching or bicycling. Swimming promotes range of motion throughout all your joints and it helps in resurfacing your joints as they become arthritic. It is one of the best exercises you can do but it does not strengthen bones.

Dancing is one of my favorite exercises because it reduces stress and promotes joint movement. While you're dancing you are moving and having fun. You are building up new bone, strengthening your bones and reducing the risk of fractures. It can be a great social experience and you can do it well into your nineties.

Single retirees rarely get to touch someone. Touch is so important to our wellbeing that infants fail to thrive unless they are constantly touched. Through dancing you get to touch someone and connect briefly. That contact with another human being makes you feel better.

Since I am a ballroom and swing dancer, I have noticed a lot of healthy people in their eighties who are dancers. The good health of older dancers led me to write my last book *Dance to Live*. This book explained the health benefits one gets by dancing. By dancing you strengthen your bones, improve your balance and your memory, get cardiovascular exercise and increase your stamina. You also have a good time while interacting socially with others. The book is an easy read and the information will convince you that dancing is one of the best forms of exercise you can have.

I saw an article recently about a ninety-eight-year-old woman in Naples, Florida, who still dances several times a week. She had an interesting motto for life: "Smile awhile and while you smile, another smiles. Soon there are miles and miles of smiles. And life is worthwhile because you smile."

You should move as much as you can to reduce the stress on your joints by weight maintenance. Caloric restriction is one of the better ways to do it. That alone will increase your life.

You should exercise your body, your mind, and at the same time eat less. If you do that, you'll have a greater chance of living longer and know that you are living well. If you stress your body through exercise, give it proper nutrients, and reduce your caloric intake, you'll have a better balance in the body's chemical reactions. Your body and mind will give you much better service.

Remember the studies I quoted with the rats who were mentally stimulated, as well as the nuns who were intellectually stimulated well into their nineties and had the brains of young people, and the ninety-year-olds who increased their muscle strength by 174%. All of this is possible. And don't forget the astronaut John Glenn who performed as well as forty-year-olds after his space flight.

Everything is possible if you get moving. What did Jack LaLane, the old guru of exercise, affirm? When he wrote his book at the age of eighty three, he said, "Old age is always twenty years away." He also stated, "There ain't no fountain of youth. What you put into your body is exactly what you get out of it." How true that is.

And that is accurate in everything. What you put into your life you get out of it. How you made your bed is exactly how you will lie in it. What you sow is exactly what you will reap.

Now for the finale: **The Lenhart exercise program for longevity.** I came up with this formula after reviewing dozens of articles on physical activity for the lectures I gave to physicians who took the anti-aging seminars. If you follow these examples, it will greatly increase your chance of living longer and healthier. As well, staying mentally alert will keep you excited about life.

1. Pump iron for 15-minutes to the point of discomfort. That means lifting various types of weights to stress and eventually build muscles. You can use free weights or the machines at the gym. I generally have the weight set where I can only do 10-15 reps. Take rest breaks between muscle groups. For aerobic exercises with machines use more reps and less weight.

2. Change the muscle group each time you weight-train. If you are doing upper body exercises one day, the next day do lower body exercises. It is not that difficult with machines and free weights to exercise most of the muscle groups in the body. You can change the angles of free weights for complex muscle groups.

Walk three miles in forty-five to sixty minutes, or to a slight sweat. Why is that important? You have to walk at a pace that actually stresses your body to a certain extent and gets your heart rate up. You have to sweat a little but not a lot. Just so you are slightly clammy. Sweating helps release toxins through the pores in your skin. It also builds up your cardiovascular fitness by increasing your heart rate and increasing your oxygenation.

Hippocrates, the father of medicine, stated "Walking is man's best medicine."

3. Use comfortable shock-absorbing walking shoes to reduce the ground-reactive forces on your joints. One of the major problems people have with jogging or running is that they destroy their hips, knees or ankles. I strongly recommend walking with cushioned shoes to reduce joint stress that can eventually lead to osteoarthritis. I do not feel it is necessary to run to exhaustion and destroy your joints at the same time.

It is also important to swing your arms while walking. Your left arm swings forward as you step on your right leg and vice-versa. This cross crawl pattern is important for circulation and the nervous system.

4. Smile and think happy thoughts while you are exercising. It is very important to have a good mental attitude and positive mindset most of the time. Based upon many observations, people who have the best mental attitude seem to do better later in life.

5. Constantly stimulate your mind by learning. Your mental stimulation should also be varied; the diversity of things you learn stimulates different parts of your brain. Stress your mind by learning about a subject that you know nothing about. Crossword puzzles also work.

6. Do the above exercise combinations at least three times per week.

John P. Lenhart M.D.

By the way, to exercise in an airplane, stretch your legs out and pump your feet up and down to increase your circulation and tone your muscles. If an airplane has something in front of your feet so that you can't stretch your legs out, ask to change your seat. I flew in an airplane from Europe once and the plane had an electronics box in front of my feet so I complained. The flight attendant looked for an empty seat and changed my seat. If any aeronautical engineer is reading this book, do not design airplanes that limit passengers' abilities to stretch out their legs in front of them.

Exercise is work, but the rewards are well worth it.

You may not only add years to your life, but you will add quality of life to your years.

CHAPTER 6

Vitamins, Minerals, Herbs and Anti-Oxidants

(Warning – parts of this chapter are very detailed, may be skimmed for their general meaning, and can be read in small snippets. The detailed description of vitamins is included for those individuals wanting to know more.)

In Nature, everything affects everything else. If you take one component out of the system, the entire downstream process is affected. Nature has created a balance through millions of years of adaptation. If that balance is disrupted our biological ecosystem gets thrown out of sync and may begin to self-destruct.

Sometimes our bodies can accommodate to changes and sometimes they can't. The ability to accommodate is based on our genetic makeup and our diet. The male deer in Shenandoah National Park get selected for breeding by the females by the size of their antlers. The size of their antlers is determined by their genetic makeup and the diet that they have eaten. A healthy nutritious diet will assure antler bone growth of up to a quarter inch per day. If they have a poor diet, their antlers will not grow as much and the females will not select them. They will not be able to propagate their genes.

The food we eat has the same effect on us. It has to be nutritious, with adequate vitamins and minerals in trace amounts in order for us, and our offspring, to thrive and stay healthy. As yet, doctors do not know exactly what is needed in trace amounts for optimum health and how everything interacts.

If you were stranded on a tropical island and you had the opportunity to take only a few vitamins or nutrients with you, which would you take to give you the greatest protective effect and let you live in a healthy way?

Most people would probably say vitamin C and that would be a good choice. However, on a tropical island, you would most likely have plenty of fruits. Fruits are, generally, fairly high in vitamin C, so you would get all the vitamin C you needed.

So, what would you take? How about Coenzyme Q-10? Have you ever considered that? Coenzyme Q-10 is one of the components in the energy transfer cycle in our body. This coenzyme may be an important factor when you start running out of steam and body parts start wearing out.

Getting enough Vitamin E is difficult through a normal diet. Since Vitamin E is such an important antioxidant, I would probably sneak some E along.

You may also consider taking some Alpha-Lipoic Acid along. This natural component of your cells is essential for recirculating and balancing other antioxidants which are protective in cell destruction, and it may also help cure your liver if you develop liver disease. In Germany, it is used to decrease blood sugar levels in diabetics, so if you were a non-insulin dependent diabetic with high blood sugar, you would probably want to take some of it along. It would take eating 200 lbs of spinach to give you a 100 mg tablet of Alpha-Lipoic Acid. Just in case your joints wear out, you could also keep some chondroitin and glucosamine in your bag.

John P. Lenhart M.D.

Vitamin C

I guess we will start with the most famous of the vitamins, one which probably gives you the biggest bang for the buck. Going back in my memory banks, I remember when I was a resident studying this vitamin. Even then I was very much interested in natural approaches towards healing. I would see these severely emaciated patients come in. Some were very old and had a large number of pressure sores and ulcerations around their bodies. The open sores left the patients exposed to massive infections, which would lead to death fairly rapidly. These people were sent to the rehabilitative center after being in a regular hospital, progressively getting worse due to their lack of nutrient reserves. Whenever they were laid on a bed, their skin broke down and became ulcerated.

The standard treatment, at the time, was force-feeding them Ensure, a chemical nutrient formula designed to sustain life. We fed some of them through a tube in their throat, and in others, a tube was embedded through their abdominal wall. The results were not as satisfying as I had hoped.

I started looking into vitamin C. In the medical library, I found a 1930s book about vitamin C which used all the research performed from the turn of the century to the 1930s. I was amazed at the wealth of information that existed on this vitamin so many years ago, and shocked that the medical community rarely utilized this information in their treatment protocols.

Medicine knew long ago that ascorbic acid (vitamin C) could prevent scurvy, a disease that caused the deaths of many sailors on long voyages as their diet was short on essential nutrients. However, medicine rarely used the basic scientific information that was available, as early as 1920, in treatment protocols.

Perhaps this material was ignored in part because drug companies became powerful and infectious diseases had a priority in research; as well, the business aspect of medicine became driven by drugs and high-tech surgery.

After presenting the data to my supervisors, I started an intravenous drip with vitamin C in high concentrations. I did that on a daily basis. To the surprise of the nursing staff, the severely debilitated patients began to improve fairly rapidly. Their open lesions healed and their pressure sores reduced in size.

As well, I had read some of the research done by Linus Pauling and his theory of vitamin C. I learned that he was taking about 12 to 14 grams of vitamin C per day. (Personally, I take higher doses of Vitamin C in a powdered form mixed in orange or cranberry juice along with multivitamins and vitamin E, if I feel I'm getting a little under the weather.)

The reason I gave the patients vitamin C was because I also knew it was essential for collagen formation, which is the connective component of the skin and gives the skin elasticity. When we don't have that elasticity, the skin becomes very thin and breaks down. This elasticity is necessary for all our organs.

There is a condition called scleroderma where patients' skin and connective tissue become very hard and eventually they can't move their hands. Their facial skin becomes really firm, and eventually their digestive tract and swallowing mechanism become impaired so they can't swallow.

At the time when I was giving intravenous vitamin C to my patients, I didn't know of its importance as an antioxidant and as a fighter of free radicals. Consequently, when that data emerged, intravenous vitamin C became an important component in the chelation therapy regimen.

Linus Pauling demonstrated the beneficial effect of high-dose vitamin C. I understand that he was mentally clear and in good health until his death in his nineties. He also rarely suffered from infectious diseases because he had a fairly strong immune system. His book, *Vitamin C and the Common Cold,* became a classic and popularized the use of vitamin C for preventative reasons.

When Dr. Denham Harman in 1954 came up with the theory of free radicals and described it fully, vitamin C started taking on a very important role as an antioxidant and nutrient.

As we get older, we slowly shrivel up and bake ourselves to death, like a plum in an oven that becomes a prune, or a chicken that turns brown as it bakes. Our skin slowly gets browner, gets more spots, discolors, gets cancer cells, and shrivels up.

This slow damage is caused by free radicals and the oxidation reactions that gradually destroy us.

Oxidation occurs throughout the entire environment. It is evident as rust on metal or as white powder on aluminum. Metal, if it oxidizes enough, eventually breaks down completely. Just leave a piece of metal exposed to the elements and you will witness it rust and fall apart before your eyes.

However, if you apply phosphoric acid to the metal, the rust is changed biochemically into a coating that protects the metal.

When I was at Anse-aux-Meadows, Newfoundland, where the Vikings established a colony 500 years before Columbus discovered America, I noticed that the blacksmith shop made a lot of iron nails for their ships' hulls. The nails that held the wood planks together had to be constantly coated with tar and eventually replaced because they rusted, or oxidized. With rusty nails, the Viking boats would fall apart so they had to do preventative maintenance.

If the Vikings did preventative maintenance 1000 years ago, shouldn't we at least be thinking about it also for ourselves?

In the human biological system, you add antioxidants, which inhibit the oxidative reactions occurring to your body. The more antioxidants you take, and the greater variety you have, theoretically, the slower will be your aging because you will not shrivel up as rapidly internally, or externally.

Vitamin C in high concentrations is also a chelating agent and helps bind toxic metals in our systems, just like EDTA (ethylenediamine tetra-acetic acid) does. In higher concentrations, it has a double effect of decreasing oxidation, keeping us from rusting and shriveling, and eliminating waste. A friend of mine used high dose Vitamin C in powdered form as a laxative, because in high dosages it will cause loose stools.

So what are some of the other benefits attributed to vitamin C based on research data? Vitamin C helps produce collagen, which makes connective tissue stronger. It is known as the cellular glue, and it keeps our tissues from falling apart. One good example, given earlier, is of the British sailors aboard ships who developed scurvy. Their symptoms were spongy gums, loose teeth, and bleeding into the skin and mucous membranes. Their cellular connective substance, the glue that holds all our tissues together, broke apart.

The sailors literally fell apart and bled to death because they lacked the cellular connective substance, which is essential and dependent on vitamin C. They also would have died suddenly of cardiac death because Vitamin C is also essential for heart function.

With increased vitamin C, this cellular connective substance builds a stronger connective tissue, making the body more resistant to a large host of organisms. A number of studies have demonstrated the benefits of high doses of vitamin C and its ability to fight against cancer of the mouth, throat, larynx, stomach, bladder, pancreas, breasts, skin, cervix, colon, rectum, and so on. This anti-cancer effect was well documented in Dr. Linus Pauling's book, *Cancer and Vitamin C.*

In 2015 The National Cancer Institute stated on its web site that:

- Vitamin C is a nutrient found in food and dietary supplements. It is an antioxidant and also plays a key role in making collagen .
- High-dose vitamin C may be given by intravenous (IV) infusion (through a vein into the bloodstream) or orally (taken by mouth). When taken by intravenous infusion, vitamin C can reach much higher levels in the blood than when the same amount is taken by mouth.
- High-dose vitamin C has been studied as a treatment for patients with cancer since the 1970s.
- Laboratory studies have shown that high doses of vitamin C may slow the growth and spread of prostate, pancreatic, liver, colon, and other types of cancer cells.
- Some laboratory and animal studies have shown that combining vitamin C with anticancer therapies may be helpful, while other studies have shown that certain forms of vitamin C may make chemotherapy less effective.
- Animal studies have shown that high-dose vitamin C treatment blocks tumor growth in certain models of pancreatic, liver, prostate, and ovarian cancers, sarcoma, and malignant mesothelioma.
- Some human studies of high-dose IV vitamin C in patients with cancer have shown improved quality of life, as well as improvements in physical, mental, and emotional functions, symptoms of fatigue, nausea and vomiting, pain, and appetite loss.
- Intravenous high-dose ascorbic acid has caused very few side effects in clinical trials.
- While generally approved as a dietary supplement, the U.S. Food and Drug Administration (FDA) has not approved the use of IV high-dose vitamin C as a treatment for cancer or any other medical condition.

The details of its process are beyond the scope of this book, other than to make you aware that vitamin C is an extremely potent protector of our connective tissues. It neutralizes a number of carcinogens, including pesticides, nitrites, nitrosamines, hydrocarbons, air pollutants, industrial chemicals, and so forth. Remember, as I told you earlier, vitamin C in high doses is also a potent chelating agent. It helps remove toxic elements from your body.

Another benefit of vitamin C is that it enhances T-lymphocytes, which are the blood components in the immune system that help to kill cancer cells. The stronger your immune system, the greater your ability to fight a large host of organisms. Vitamin C has also been found to be beneficial to people with cataracts and has helped prevent cataracts in rats. Asthma symptoms have also been reduced by the intake of vitamin C supplementation.

The intensity and frequency of common colds are both reduced when one takes high doses of vitamin C, as exhibited by Dr. Linus Pauling.

Sperm quality, especially in heavy smokers, has been improved by higher dosages of vitamin C. In a 2006 research article, sperm count was increased and sperm mobility was significantly increased by taking 1000 mgs of vitamin C twice daily for 2 months. Vitamin C has shown anti-candida effect. Serum cholesterol has dropped with administrations of one gram of vitamin C. Platelet adhesiveness and platelet aggregation have been decreased with vitamin C, therefore reducing blood clotting.

Other studies showed that six weeks of vitamin C supplementation lowered pulse and systolic blood pressure in patients with borderline hypertension. A Japanese study in terminal cancer patients showed a survival time that was up to five times longer among patients given vitamin C than among the non-vitamin C patients.

The evidence goes on and on with a host of worldwide studies showing the benefits of vitamin C.

As revealed, vitamin C is an effective immune enhancing agent, increasing your resistance. It is a potent scavenger of free radicals, which cause you to age and shrivel away.

The studies on vitamin C are too numerous to elaborate, but the data have been available since the thirties when the original studies were made on guinea pigs, with the promotion of wound healing by the use of vitamin C and its requirement for collagen synthesis. The free radical and anti-aging benefits of vitamin C have only recently been recognized since free radicals have been identified in our aging and disease processes.

For how many years have you heard "sunscreen, sunscreen, sunscreen" for the prevention of skin cancers, some of which could be deadly? In a recent meeting of the American College of Dermatology, new findings came to light. Although the American population had been using high amounts of sunscreen, the skin cancer rate remained the same or *increased*. If sunscreens were to protect against skin cancer, they certainly didn't do a good job. It appears that all they managed to do was protect against sunburn.

The newest theory is that free radical damage to our skin actually caused the cancer. Now they recommend high dosages of antioxidants, including multiple servings of fruits and vegetables daily. I find that to be an interesting shift in focus from the previous chemical drugs and surgical treatment to a more preventative approach.

So, what does all this have to do with longevity?

If you have a healthy immune system and fewer diseases, you'll have a greater chance of living longer. The less ill you are, the greater will be your ability to enjoy life to its fullest, even at an old age.

Reducing free radical damage to your system, be it in the skin, brain, arterial system, plaque buildup, or cancers, will greatly enhance your chances to survive into old age. It certainly makes sense to me that vitamin C is a good preventative measure to take in your anti-aging program.

Nutrition-minded doctors recommend 1000 to 3000 mg of the ester vitamin C. I personally like taking the powdered form of vitamin C because it is easy to digest; it mixes with juice, and gives me a high dose fairly rapidly. The bioflavonoids, which are extremely important, are obtained through a multivitamin, as well as the fruits and vegetables I eat.

Vitamin E

While vitamin C is water soluble, vitamin E is a fat-soluble vitamin. There are eight different forms of Vitamin E: alpha, beta, gamma, and delta-tocopherol; and also alpha, beta, gamma, and delta-tocotrienol. These will be explained further on. Vitamin E is just as important an antioxidant as vitamin C. Vitamins E and C seem to work together to enhance antioxidant benefits as well as in increasing resistance. Vitamin C is essential in improving your immune function, increasing your T- and B-lymphocytes, which are essential for your immunity.

The saturated fats that we eat in our diet are oxidized into free radicals. The antioxidant properties of vitamin E help prevent that process, thereby reducing our oxidative stress, and may reduce our chance of getting various cancers, such as colon or breast. This is a complex subject with no definitive answers as yet, because vitamins work in combinations. Taking one specific vitamin in a trial may not give you any results. If you ate just one food, you would probably get sick because you need a variety of vitamins, trace minerals, fats and protein for overall health.

I usually take 800 I.U. all natural vitamin E without oil fillers. Oil fillers are found in the synthetic vitamin E, which is mostly alpha d-tocopherol. Based on various experiments, just taking alpha d-tocopherol suppresses the natural gamma tocopherol, and after a while depletes it from your body, but gamma tocopherol has a sparing effect on alpha tocopherol, keeping it from being depleted. Gamma tocopherol is very protective of your body and helps keep your blood thinner. Warning – more than 1,000 mg/day or 1,500 IU/day of synthetic Vitamin E may cause uncontrolled bleeding in some people. Talk to your doctor first.

There's a big difference in pricing between the cheap, synthetic tocopherols and the all-natural, pure vitamin E mixed tocopherol. It is thought that with the mixed tocopherols, the natural vitamin E complex, you get the anti-thrombotic (less tendency for your blood to clot) function of d-alpha and d-gamma tocopherol along with antioxidant properties of d-beta, d-gamma, and d-delta tocopherols, which help protect you from the harmful free radicals.

You may also want to check what type of gelatin capsule they use for the vitamin E. The bovine is thought to be better than the porcine, especially with people who have difficulty with pork products. You see, the cheap vitamin E may have soy or other oil fillers, which may, after a prolonged period, turn rancid even inside the capsules and cause their own free radical problems.

Some of you may be saying, "Whoa, I didn't understand anything you said."

Let me break it down: Anti-thrombotic means it decreases the ability of getting blood clots. It means it helps reduce the thrombosis, the clot formation. Blood clots can be very dangerous. They can stop your lungs from oxygenating. They can migrate up to the brain and cause you to have a stroke. They can get stuck in your legs and cause you to have deep venous thrombosis and pain in the legs, as well as intermittent claudication, the periodic obstruction of blood supply to the legs. A clot can also suddenly form in your heart causing a sudden heart attack without warning. Cardiologists generally recommend a baby aspirin daily to thin your blood and help prevent blood clots.

I mentioned the antioxidant component of vitamin E when I talked about vitamin C properties. The antioxidant action helps neutralize the harmful free radicals which cause disease, induce cellular damage and aging itself. A good test is to cut an apple in half and squeeze some lemon juice on one half and nothing on the other half. Cover both halves with cellophane, if you want, and watch what happens to the color. The lemon juice acts as an anti-oxidant and keeps the cut apple from turning brown.

Remember, the more antioxidants you have in your system, the better you are protected.

One word of caution about vitamin E: Because vitamin E has a tendency to thin your blood you should avoid vitamin E prior to any surgery. Talk to your doctor about vitamin E and Coumadin, if you are taking it (since Coumadin also thins your blood).

The antioxidant action of vitamin E is synergistic with vitamin C. The two, along with other antioxidants, are essential to keep free radicals from destroying your body fairly rapidly. You see, there is a finely tuned checks-and-balances system between free radical damage and free radical protection and repair.

With our increased consumption of free radical producing foods, and our environment worsened by the thousands of chemicals and radiation we are exposed to, high dosages of antioxidants may help maintain cellular balance and keep things from falling apart.

Free radicals produce a tremendous amount of stress in our bodies. The more junk we are exposed to in our environment and food, the greater the free radical damage. Therefore, you need high concentrations of these anti free radical antioxidants along with plenty of fruits and vegetables to mitigate the damage as much as possible.

Look at it this way, the higher your stress level, the greater your need for stress reduction techniques and relaxation.

As well, Vitamin E is very useful to the reproductive system. Tocopherol is a Greek word for "the ability to reproduce." Numerous studies have shown that vitamin E also increases your stamina level and reduces your fatigue level.

Dr. Wilfrid Shute, a prominent vitamin E researcher, demonstrated the benefits of vitamin E for energy. Other studies in Czechoslovakia and

Russia confirm the benefits of vitamin E in increased athletic performance.

As early as the 1920s, vitamin E was used to enhance the fertility of animals. Lack of vitamin E in their diet caused a shriveling of their sexual organs. Another report indicates that vitamin E may help prevent miscarriages by helping the placenta imbed itself into the uterus.

Vitamin E helps prevent platelet aggregation so there is greater blood flow, without obstruction, to various important sexual organs that enhance sexual pleasure. Vitamin E and the sex hormones are chemically related.

Numerous other benefits have been attributed to vitamin E, including healing wounds of the skin, reducing scars, repairing skin burn damage, and reducing wrinkles, especially stretch marks after pregnancy.

Vitamin E has been used for a long time for prevention of cardiovascular problems, including transient ischemic attacks (TIAs) or minor strokes. One study compared results of vitamin E plus aspirin with aspirin by itself. The findings showed that there was a significant reduction in the rate of TIAs in the vitamin E plus aspirin group.

This makes sense because we know that vitamin E decreases the stickiness of platelets, as does aspirin. You're getting double the amount of anti-platelet activity, which decreases small clots, thereby decreasing the mini-stroke level.

One of the biggest problems occurring in society today is the prevalence of Alzheimer's disease. I mentioned that fact, previously, in the physical activity section in this book, and also in the detoxification section.

Alzheimer's patients have a high level of amyloid beta protein, which accumulates over a period of time and sludges up the brain cells. Vitamin

E seems to inhibit this amyloid beta protein, a key component seen in brain cell death that leads to progressive memory loss.

One interesting finding I discovered from my old literature sources was a degeneration or dystrophy of voluntary muscles that occurred in virtually all animals that had been deprived of vitamin E. Also, years ago, they discovered that muscular dystrophy occurred in vitamin E deficient children.

I looked at data from books written in the 1940s, which described in detail the benefits of vitamin E based on clinical observations. Unfortunately, the benefits described in these old texts were never seized upon by the medical world because there were no double-blind clinical trials for many of these observations.

Years ago people thought drugs would solve everything. Well, they didn't. Drugs became a crutch for disease, not a solution for it. People have become dependent on drugs for survival. The emphasis in medicine has been on drug treatment for symptoms of disease (the focus of most physicians), rather than prevention of the disease. In ancient China, the Chinese paid their doctors to keep them healthy and if they got sick the doctor had to treat them for free.

Of course, for North Americans, many of our practices have been driven by the profit potential of the drugs themselves. Do you realize that it was not until 1959 that the Food and Drug Administration recognized that vitamin E was essential? It was not until 1968 that they came out with a recommended minimum daily requirement.

In 1971, a medical publication stated that vitamin E had no value for any human ailment, yet recommendations were made in 1973 for adding vitamin E to infant formulas. Also, at that time, it was noted that vitamin E might be of benefit for intermittent claudication (calf pain due to poor circulation while walking). As in the 1971 publication, the December, 2013 *Annals of Internal Medicine* published three articles indicating that vitamin and mineral supplements for the general population were a waste of money. Their opinion was based on analysis of a variety of studies. (This reminds me of the period when everyone had their tonsils removed because they were considered useless organs, and now that we understand the immune system better, we recognize their importance.)

Additionally, Vitamin E is closely linked with selenium for antibody production. Studies have shown, based upon control groups, that animals given selenium had a twelve percent increase in antibody production; however, those given selenium plus vitamin E doubled in antibody production. Note again the benefits of vitamin E in immune function.

Selenium is an important trace metal, which should be included in your prevention regimen. People with low selenium intake have been associated with higher rates of cancer deaths.

Studies completed in 1973, using Vitamin E and selenium in conjunction revealed a reduction of angina pectoris. It was later reported that veterinarians had been using vitamin E long before for reducing symptoms of angina in animals.

Vitamin E has also reduced damage and given a protective effect to chromosomes, induced from free radical inducing radiation and other carcinogens.

While researching older literature sources, I found studies revealing that vitamin E reduced the incidence of cancer in animals that had been force-fed known carcinogens versus the control group. An interesting finding, don't you think?

There are numerous benefits to vitamins E and C combined, such as relief of pain from osteoarthritis and protection from light-induced cataracts in animals. Vitamin E also helps provide protection from the pain caused by anoxic (lack of oxygen) damage.

Neurological disorders caused by lack of oxygen improved when vitamin E was supplemented. In a Vitamin E study for moderately severe

Alzheimer's patients, a lower number of those taking Vitamin E became incapacitated, over a two year period, compared to the placebo group.

Now for the negative study: There was a 2005 meta-analysis (a review of many previous studies) in the *Annals of Internal Medicine* which concluded that high dose vitamin E, greater than 400IU, increased all-cause mortality. However, it also said that the studies reviewed for high dose vitamin E were small and done on patients with chronic diseases. It also stated that, "The generalizability of the findings to healthy adults is uncertain." That last line didn't make the news. When you look into these reports you have to look into the details, and no mention was made as to what kind of Vitamin E was used nor how sick the patients were.

However, in 2014, a study published in the *Journal of the American Medical Association* found that among patients with mild to moderate Alzheimer's Disease (AD), those given 2000 IU/d of alpha-tocopherol (vitamin E), compared with the placebo patients, resulted in slower functional decline. There were no significant differences in the groups receiving memantine alone or memantine plus alpha-tocopherol. "These findings suggest benefit of alpha-tocopherol in mild to moderate AD by slowing functional decline and decreasing caregiver burden." If you can delay progression of Alzheimer's Disease by 6 months, that's a huge savings to the health care system.

In the January 2011 publication of *Reproductive Health*, Brazilian researchers, using a supplement containing 1 or 2 grams of vitamin E and essential fatty acids, reported that the combination may help reduce symptoms of premenstrual syndrome (PMS). The women showed marked improvements in their PMS symptoms at six months, compared to women who received a placebo. The greatest improvement was seen in the higher dose supplement.

Earlier, Vitamin E was thought to protect men from prostate cancer. However, based on the SELET trial (Selenium and Vitamin E cancer prevention trial) initiated in 2001 with 35,000 men, using the dl-alpha-tocopherol component of vitamin E, prostate cancer increased. (Note that the natural form is d-alpha-tocopherol and not dl-alpha-tocopherol that was used in the study.) The results were published in JAMA 2009.

The results concluded that men taking 400 IU of the dl-alpha-tocopherol vitamin E had a 17% higher occurrence of prostate cancer than among men taking a placebo. (However, they did not use the entire Vitamin E molecule in nature which has alpha, beta and gamma components.) Additionally, the National Cancer Institute reported in 2014 that men with high levels of selenium at the start of the trial had double the chance of developing prostate cancer. The study was undertaken because previous data showed that vitamin E plus selenium might reduce prostate cancer.

This was a huge trial. What bothers me is why they didn't use the natural d-alpha form of vitamin E? The synthetic dl-alpha-tocopherol vitamin E is the cheap form available everywhere. Synthetic vitamin E may have a different effect on our bodies than the natural form.

As revealed earlier, there are eight different forms of Vitamin E: alpha, beta, gamma, and delta-tocopherol; and also alpha, beta, gamma, and delta-tocotrienol. Alpha-tocopherol is the most active form in humans.

The Linus Pauling Institute Micronutrient Information Center, at the Oregon State University, is an excellent source for Vitamin information. Their web site publishes the significant studies done on Vitamin E, as well as on other vitamins. There is conflicting data out there. Ninety percent of men and women in the USA do not meet the minimum daily requirement of vitamin E 15mg/d 22.5 IU. On average, Americans consume 6.9 mg/d, according to the 2003-2006 *National Health and Nutrition Examination Survey.*

Based on the recent data, high dose vitamin E benefits are inconclusive for chronic diseases and some studies using dl-alpha-tocopherol show harm.

Smoking produces a considerable amount of free radical damage to the body. Vitamin E, along with vitamin C, has been shown to be helpful in reducing that damage.

People with intermittent claudication taking vitamin E appear to have less symptoms and decreased leg pain when they walk.

You may also consider taking Tocotrienols which are precursors of Vitamin E. Tocotrienols have been shown to have an effect on breast cancer cells, to break chain reactions of free radicals and to have stabilized carotid stenosis lesions. They have also decreased total cholesterol-- lowered LDL cholesterol and increased HDL cholesterol (the good cholesterol).

As you can see, vitamin E has a very important role in your anti-aging regimen. Probably the most important role is that of its antioxidant properties, in combination with vitamin C. Recent data, however, indicate that high dosages are not effective for certain conditions and may be dangerous in some cases.

When you can neutralize the free radical damage to your body, you are, in effect, lessening the aging process. When you can walk better, you have a greater quality of life. When you have less chest pain, more energy, and a healthy relationship, you are increasing your quality of life.

Remember, anti-aging is trying to recoup your physiological state, that is, the state your body performed at when it was much younger.

Beta-Carotene

With an abundance of vitamins and minerals available, it can be difficult to determine which is the most beneficial. Beta-carotene, a vitamin A precursor, stands right up there with vitamins C and E.

Free radicals cause your body to become stiff and hard, like rawhide, through a process known as crossed linking of protein strands. This crossed linking and hardening of tissues is associated with many signs of aging, such as wrinkles, cataracts, and arterial sclerosis (the hardening of your arteries).

With large consumption of antioxidants, you can neutralize free radicals and eventually turn them into water. Beta carotene inhibits LDL cholesterol (the bad cholesterol), increases oxidation and thereby might decrease the risk of heart disease. It also may be preventive in breast cancer. It is also protective to the skin and may help prevent cancerous lesions of the skin.

Beta-carotene is depleted in people who have a lot of ultraviolet exposure. That depletion leads to increased free radical damage due to the radiation.

There are numerous animal studies showing the beneficial effects of beta-carotene, or beta-carotene in combination with vitamin A and/or retinoic acid, in the prevention of various cancers. I found another study in which rats, with induced arthritis, had a decrease in arthritic symptoms after taking beta-carotene.

There is a disease, called photodermatosis, which makes people sensitive to any type of sunlight. As highlighted in a study, after subjects took beta-carotene, their tolerance increased threefold.

The retinoids, (which include retinol, retinal, isotretinoin, alitretinoin and tretinoin – Retin-A the pharmaceutical form of retinoic acid) are active components of vitamin A. They are important in vision, growth of bone, immune function, and activation of tumor suppressor genes. As a class they have been shown to be protective against a number of cancers including those of the larynx, esophagus, prostate, colon, skin, rectum, bladder, breast, stomach, lung, and cervix.

Tretinoin helps the skin renew itself. It has been used to treat acne and in the reduction of fine wrinkles and mottled skin discoloration. Rough facial skin can be made to feel smoother with tretinoin. Ask your dermatologist about it.

The use of all-trans retinoic acid, a recognized treatment for acute promyelocytic leukemia, has been shown to improve survival rates.

There appears to be a clinical correlation between lower levels of retinoids, vitamin A, and beta-carotene in populations with high cancer rates. Vitamin A and beta-carotene keep the antibody and T-lymphocyte levels high, protecting against carcinogens.

Did you know that once beta-carotene is inside your body it turns into retinol, an active form of vitamin A? You can tolerate relatively high amounts of beta-carotene, 50,000-100,000 IUs; however, you do have to be careful not to get too much vitamin A. If you take more than 50,000 IUs of vitamin A, you may see reversible toxicity symptoms of hypervitaminosis A. You may get bone and joint pain, fatigue, insomnia, hair loss, dryness and fissures of the lips and other tissues, anorexia, weight loss, enlarged liver, among other ailments.

You can tolerate 10,000, 20,000, or 30,000 IUs of vitamin A and beta-carotene combined, along with mixed carotenoids. Talk to your doctor first because toxicity is a possibility. One lucky thing is that beta-carotene is fairly readily available. It is prominent in red, dark green, orange, and yellow vegetables and fruits. That, in itself, is a better antioxidant than vitamin A. Vitamin A, being fat soluble and stored in the liver, is also found in eggs, milk, fish, fats, liver oils, and organ meats.

I like the cod liver oil form of vitamin A, however, halibut liver oil has a hundred times as much vitamin A concentration as cod liver oil has. The best way to take cod liver oil is when the smell is taken out of it. I get it from Norway, and my patients think it tastes fairly neutral. It has high levels of Omega-3 fatty acids, EPA and DHA along with vitamin A and vitamin D.

Beta-carotene and other food-derived carotenoids are nontoxic. Even at the equivalent of 100,000 IU a day, vitamin A given in beta-carotene form over three months, showed no increase in serum vitamin A and no toxicity. Beta-carotene conversion to vitamin A does not automatically follow absorption of beta-carotene. Beta-carotene in itself is an extremely potent free radical scavenger.

However, if you are deficient in vitamin A, you get night blindness, dry mucous membranes, bladder stones, decreased resistance to infection, itchy and burning eyes, and decreasing mucous formation in your lungs. A scarcity in mucous leads to a greater chance of infections and chemical irritations.

You may be deficient in vitamin A and not know it. Nitrates from fertilizer found in foods, livestock, and water, interfere with carotene conversion to vitamin A. So, you're losing the free radical fighting ability of this extremely important nutrient and may, as a consequence, age faster.

Vitamin A and the precursor of it, beta-carotene, are essential for smell, hearing, skin, teeth, and bone growth. A gradual decrease of that essential vitamin and its precursor can lead to deficiencies. What happens when you age? Your sense of smell decreases, your hearing gets bad, your skin turns wrinkly, your teeth start falling out, and you get osteoporotic.

One other caution. Cooking decreases vitamin A. So, too, does exposure to light, which is understandable because people with skin cancer have decreased levels of vitamin A and beta-carotene in their system, especially at the surface.

If you look at a lot of cosmetic products, they contain Retin-A or retinoic acid for good reason; that is, to protect your skin from the powerful ultraviolet rays. Years ago, I was very interested in Retin-A, and did a lot of research on it, because I thought it was a great way to make people's skin look young.

While researching Retin-A, I was surprised to uncover that older skin cells that had migrated to the surface were sometimes precancerous. However, the retinoic acid seemed to promote their expression and exfoliation, and newer, healthier cells grew in the place of those precancerous cells. "Voila," I said. "There is something to this vitamin and the retinoids which is essential."

When I wrote the first edition of this book, an article about tissue growth of stem cells caught my attention. Stem cells are the original embryonic cells from which all types of organs grow as they differentiate. It's a little hard to think of yourself as an embryo, but you know, believe it or not, you were there once.

Years ago, I took a research course at the Max Planck Institute in Germany where we did embryonic transplantation of rabbits. I was able to split the cells and transplant these embryonic forms into various animals. These experiments in the 70s were a precursor to the major cloning research that is now being done.

One interesting topic for me was the differentiation of various organ systems in the growth cycle of an embryo. When, exactly, do certain organs form? The theory was that the genetic code triggered formation of various basic organ systems, or body structures, relatively early in the embryonic development. Some parts such as the spinal cord and nervous system developed extremely early, while the extremities would develop later on.

I never gave much thought to the retinoids as being a major component in that developmental process until I read an article that flipped a switch within me and correlated all the past information I had read earlier about Retin-A and beta-carotene.

One morning, a newspaper article caught my attention about research being done at Tokyo University by Makoto Ashima. The headline was, "Scientists Grow Frog Eyes/Ears from Cells," using the animal's own embryo cells.

The key part of this article was that the embryo cells were cultivated in retinoic acid solutions for five days to produce the organs. The most interesting part was that varying the concentration of the retinoic acid somehow brings forth different genetic instructions to the cells. While a lower concentration produces eyes, a higher concentration activates genes producing ears. Again, the researchers were using embryonic stem cells.

That article hit me like a sledgehammer. It correlated much of the information I had learned over the years and helped to solidify my belief of retinoic acid, beta-carotene, and vitamin A as significant factors in the anti-aging process. That's why you're reading about it right now. Beta-carotene is a precursor of vitamin A, is nontoxic, and is an extremely potent antioxidant.

Retinoic acid, in itself, determines the differentiation of cells. It makes the skin younger. It guards against a host of aberrations, such as cancer. It keeps your cells from being destroyed, as with sun-damaged skin, and promotes new, healthy skin growth.

To return to beta-carotene the precursor of retinol, the best way to have it is to take it as a supplement in the form of mixed natural carotenoids of between 15,000 and 50,000IUs. The combination generally contains natural lipochromes such as beta-carotene, alpha-carotene, xanthein, lutein, and lycopene.

Some of the best foods containing beta-carotene besides the animal and fish products previously mentioned are asparagus, broccoli, carrots, cantaloupes, cherries, collard greens, tomatoes, turnips, yams, soy beans, prunes, peaches, persimmons, papaya, parsley, mangoes, and apricots. Just think of any vegetables and fruits that are green, orange, or yellow; they should contain fairly decent quantities of beta-carotene.

By now you probably know much more about beta-carotene and vitamin A than you ever dreamed possible. However, in selecting the most important healthy aging supplements, I felt this nutrient deserved considerable attention because the less free radical damage you have in your body, the lower are your chances of developing a large slew of age-related illnesses. You may also look and feel younger, which is the whole purpose of this book.

Many people's diets, especially for the elderly, do not contain adequate amounts and varieties of vegetables providing the source of this important nutrient. That is why I recommended supplementation in the mixed form. Just as natural vitamin E is better for you than the synthetic form, mixed carotenoids are most likely better for you than beta-carotene by itself.

Selenium

With so many herbs, vitamins, and minerals to choose from, selenium stands out as a potent antioxidant. It is part of a substance called glutathione peroxidase, which is an enzyme that prevents oxidation of fats, known as lipids, and assists regeneration and reformation of vitamin E. Studies on selenium show it helps prevent, and can treat, animal cancers.

A Dutch study on lung cancer in humans found an inverse relationship between selenium intake and the incidence of lung cancer. In other words, the less selenium you have, the higher your incidence of lung cancer.

Selenium, along with beta-carotene, has been shown to enhance the immune functions of elderly people. The best-known role of selenium is in the prevention of heart disease. Animal studies have shown that when it was added to the water of rats, the heart muscle was protected against lack of oxygenation. Other selenium studies on rabbits showed protective effects for the heart when they were fed high fat diets.

Along with enhancing the immune system, selenium ties into cancer-preventive properties. This was pointed out in studies where people who ate crops grown in selenium deficient soil, as Lima, Ohio, had the highest cancer rates. Conversely, people in Rapid City, North Dakota, who ate crops grown in high selenium soil in, had the lowest cancer rates.

Rapid City residents revealed the highest level of selenium in their blood, while the Lima population had half that amount. .

Did you know that horses are given selenium supplements with their hay on a regular basis? What do horse breeders know that doctors don't?

With the combination of vitamin E and selenium, you have a double boost of cancer protection properties. Selenium also helps to detoxify the body of impurities, such as heavy metals.

Selenium deficiencies are known to exist in patients with cardiovascular disease, cirrhosis, cancer, and older patients with arthritis.

It is very difficult to get adequate amounts of selenium in your diet. It is found in Brazil nuts, yeast, wheat germ, rice, and whole grains, such as brown rice, onions, garlic and mushrooms. There are also selenium shampoos. However, the best way to get selenium is through supplementation.

The supplementation is generally 100 mcg to 200 mcg per day. You get sodium selenite, selinate, or selenium-rich kelp. You have to be cautious about inorganic forms of selenium. Selenomethionine is often present in multivitamins.

What I like most about selenium is its antioxidant properties in the anti-aging program as well as its synergistic and regenerative reaction with vitamin E, which I consider to be one of the most important antioxidants for longevity. Selenium is also a free radical scavenger gobbling up those nasty little free radicals that zap holes in our cells.

Coenzyme Q-10 (ubiquinone)

Until recently, very few people had heard of Co-Q10. Previously, it was known primarily in biochemistry circles and by people studying organic chemistry. There is a cycle in the body called the energy cycle (Krebs cycle), and it is a biochemical cycle of interactions with specific substances that produce energy. It's like an electrical generating plant, powering the world around it. Co-Q10 resembles a cog in a wheel that transforms energy for our bodies to use, yet this internal manufacturing wheel deteriorates with age.

I highlight Co-Q10 here because without sufficient energy it is difficult to get anything done. Another name for Co-Q10 is ubiquinone. I included it for anti-aging because, over time, the amount of Co-Q10 declines. It is fat soluble and found primarily in the membranes of the mitochondria, which are the energy producers of our cells. In large concentrations, it is shown to improve heart function in patients with dying hearts, as well as helping in alleviating muscular dystrophy and other muscle disorders by supplying the necessary energy for those muscles to work.

Co-Q10 is essential in the production of ATP (adenosine triphosphate), a stored form of energy in our body. Just think of it as a transformer in the electrical system, transforming energy to be stored. We use ATP to provide energy to our body and make things move. Going back to making things move, I stated over and over again that Movement Is Life.

Co-Q10 is an important component in producing movement in our bodies. It has been helpful in combatting heart failure and high blood pressure as a potent antioxidant, like other supplements I have mentioned. It may also help in cancer protection.

Some studies have shown a decrease in the size of breast cancer tumors with Co-Q10. I have attended conferences where case studies were presented of patients dying of congestive heart failure being totally revived with high concentrations of Coenzyme Q-10, as it gave heart cells an extra boost of energy.

Higher concentrations of Co-Q10 are found in the nerves, as well as the heart, brain, and liver (the main detoxifier in our body). You can see that these all require large concentrations of energy to function, as does our brain to think, making Coenzyme Q-10 a very important anti-aging substance.

Most important of all, it helps to protect us against free radicals. You may notice I keep harping on about free radicals. Well, it is extremely important. Anything that helps fight free radical production helps us age less.

Conditions that have been treated with Co-Q10 include senility, infertility, low sperm count, and periodontal disease, as well as ringing of the ears. It seems to also help regulate the immune system.

There are a host of studies showing the benefits of Co-Q10 on the heart muscle, from fighting against cardiomyopathy to congestive heart failure to arrhythmias. It also appears to help heart cell damage during bypass surgery. Animal studies have shown anti-cancer effects of Co-Q10. Breast cancer patients have also received benefits from Co-Q10.

As I mentioned, Co-Q10 is important in the energy cycle. As we grow older, our energy levels decrease and so does the level of Co-Q10.

You generally don't need Co-Q10 if you're younger than thirty. However, the body is genetically programmed to decrease production of Co-Q10 as you get older. After age thirty, the production of Co-Q10 declines and you are more prone to oxidative damage. Coenzyme Q-10 is found in seafood, meats, and whole grains.

The daily dosage of Co-Q10 is from 50 to 600 mg per day. The higher dosages are used for therapeutic effects. At the higher dosages, 300 mg or more, taken in divided doses, people have noticed a higher energy state.

You have to be cautious with Co-Q10 because it has been known to decrease the action of Coumadin, a blood thinner.

B12, B6, and Other B Vitamins

Here's a question for you. Why are B vitamins important in longevity? They're not really antioxidants. They don't prevent free radical damage like the other vitamins and minerals I've mentioned. So why not relegate them to the multivitamin and multimineral complex and just tell you to take them as part of your daily supplement routine?

The reason I didn't do that is because as you get older the deficiency of these vitamins (especially of B12, due to its depletion in your body), can cause such severe debilitation that you can end up with considerable neurological damage, incontinence, lethargy, and immobility. Vegetarians often lack B12 because it is not readily available in their diet. Standard laboratory tests can show that there is nothing wrong with you other than the progressively rapid onset of dementia, rigidity, immobility, and incontinence. However, if you do a B vitamin level test, you may find that you are dangerously low in B12.

How can that happen in normal, apparently healthy, individuals as they age? It is because their ability to absorb B12 diminishes over time. The microvilli, those little finger-like projections inside your intestines, become sluggish and, after a while, have a difficult time absorbing this essential nutrient. A perfectly normal, functioning, active, vigorous individual, completely in charge of his or her life that becomes depleted of B12 can turn into a basket case within a week.

A few years ago, one of my retired doctor friends started to fall and needed a cane to steady herself. After reading books on vitamins and nutrition, she started taking Vitamin B12. Slowly her balance improved and she can now walk without a cane. It's amazing how the lack of absorption of one specific vitamin can have such a devastating effect on a nervous system. (I will talk about the gut biome later on in this book.)

B vitamins are so essential to longevity that they deserve special mention. There was a case in Florida of a man charged with killing his wife. He had become delirious and demented. His excuse was vitamin B12 deficiency. He was released and reunited with his children after blood levels indicated he was, indeed, severely depleted of this essential vitamin. There have been other cases where symptoms of dementia and delirium were resolved with vitamin B12 injections.

B12, also known as cyanocobalamin, is essential for red blood-cell formation as well as in the functioning of the central nervous system, the brain and spinal cord. It also maintains fertility and helps many patients with fatigue and depression.

One reason people feel and act better with B12 (usually given as injections), is that the vitamin may be important in the production of neurotransmitters in your brain (which allow you to think and make decisions). Your mood, therefore, can be affected, as can your overall psychological well-being. It has also been used in the treatment of patients with Alzheimer's disease. As well, enhanced cognitive performance and some anti-tumor effects in mice have been revealed. Vitamin B12 also helps coat the nerve sheaths, called myelin, and aids with the overall integrity of the nervous system. The most common usage of B12 over the years has been for pernicious anemia, which is B12 anemia.

Another beneficial use of B12 is the potential to reverse some of the detrimental effects of chronic exposure to nitric oxide inhalation, an anesthetic used for dental surgery.

Multiple sclerosis patients also showed some benefits with B12 use, as did hepatitis patients. Elderly patients with low B12 levels displayed suppressed immunoglobulin levels, which is part of the immune system, and returned to normal after B12 supplementation.

Many patients come in for a B12 injection because they are fatigued or somewhat depressed. Although there is no obvious deficiency of the vitamin, they feel better after the injection. It was routinely included in my chelation vitamin drip for patients who were trying to detoxify themselves and increase their circulation.

One reason vegetarians may become deficient in vitamin B12 is that it is principally found in animal food products, such as fish, meat, eggs, and dairy. Most multivitamins contain B12. Boosters of 1000 mcg are often given intramuscularly or intravenously to help people feel better.

Vitamin B6, also known as pyridoxine, has also been extensively studied. Many consider B6 to be one of the most important B vitamins. It is an essential component in the metabolism of fats, carbohydrates, potassium, iron, adrenaline, insulin, and protein. You need B6 for the absorption of amino acids, which are found in protein, and also in the synthesis of antibodies, as well as DNA and RNA, the programming codes of your cells.

One problem with B6 is that it is very easily destroyed in food processing. As with B12 deficiencies, B6 deficiencies can cause nerve problems, seizures, intestinal problems, neuropathy (when nerves die), and various forms of edema. B6 combined with folic acid has been shown to reduce heart disease.

Patients usually take anywhere from 2 to 300 mg. Generally, you can find it in liver and other meats, as well as in wheat.

I emphasize B6 because it, too, is important in the manufacturing of neurotransmitters and the maintaining of mental function as you get older. Memory has been improved in elderly individuals who were given 20 mg of B6 for three months. B6 has also been used in the treatment of autistic children.

In dosages of 100 to 150 mg per day, B6 has helped relieve some of the symptoms of carpal tunnel syndrome. It also has improved symptoms of PMS (premenstrual syndrome), as well as nausea and vomiting during pregnancy.

B6 is included in the anti-aging vitamins because elderly patients are often anemic and need to be supplemented with both B6 and B12. Vitamin B6 also helps with protein metabolism and with the integrity of the nervous system. This is important because as one ages decreased nervous system response is evident.

The other B vitamins that are often found in B complex supplements, are also essential, such as B1 (thiamine), which is involved in sugar metabolism and prevention of neuritis, anxiety, fatigue, and irritability. Similarly, Riboflavin, which is B2, is important for protein metabolism and tissue repair. It helps convert the amino acid tryptophan to niacin, also known as B3.

Niacin deficiency causes the 4 D's--dementia, diarrhea, dermatitis, and death. Niacin deficiency is also associated with cold legs and arms, fatigue, and headaches.

Folic acid, another type of B vitamin, is important for red blood cell formation and synthesis of DNA, the building blocks of our bodies. It helps with repairing tissues.

Vitamin B5 (pantothenic acid) is essential in the synthesis of fatty acids and is a precursor of cholesterol and adrenal hormones. It also helps in heme formation, which is part of hemoglobin, part of our red blood cells.

If you don't have enough pantothenic acid, you can suffer fatigue, decreased appetite, constipation, increased infection, decreased blood pressure, and so on. Another important aspect of pantothenic acid is that it is actually involved in the energy production cycle known as the Krebs cycle, just as is Coenzyme Q-10. It is part of a substance called acetyl/coenzyme A, which starts the whole cycle going.

Some of these details may be beyond your interest, but I included them to show you the importance of Vitamin B5 in longevity and in the prevention of neurological and blood problems, which occur as you age.

Many of the elderly patients I have seen have shown a gradual decrease in their nervous system ability as well as in their red blood cell production with, at times, chronic anemia. You may recall the study done of the oldest man in Japan, that was mentioned earlier, who had similar symptoms. .

It is clear from this discussion that supplementation of B vitamins is essential in any longevity program.

Ginkgo Biloba

The ginkgo tree, native to Asia, is one of the world's oldest living trees. As a matter of fact, the ginkgo tree can live up to 4,000 years and is extremely resilient.   It can withstand environmental pollutants and diseases that have destroyed many other tree species.

Ginkgo biloba extract is made from the leaves and is found to be a potent antioxidant and circulation enhancer, especially in small blood vessels.

As we age, blood vessels gradually become clogged. The more clogged they become, the less circulation occurs and the less oxygen and fewer nutrients reach your blood cells. This circulatory decline can also affect the connective nerve fibers between different areas of the brain and spinal cord.

With decreased circulation to the nerve fibers, you have decreased ability of the nerves to make connections with one another, thereby decreasing your ability to make rational decisions and think clearly.

Ginkgo biloba increases circulation, allowing the nerve endings to better connect. Also, it provides for the nourishment of the small cells in your brain with rich life-sustaining oxygen and nutrients. With this boost of nutrients and oxygen, your mental performance may increase to near normal levels and the deficits normally seen with aging are greatly diminished. Signs of dementia and senility may also improve, allowing you to become yourself again.

Studies have shown ginkgo biloba to improve memory and reduce depression, headaches, tinnitus and leg cramps. It has lowered blood pressure in individuals and decreased platelet clumping, which can lead to strokes.

Ginkgo is now being used for treatment of Alzheimer's disease because it has been shown to improve memory and alertness in some people. People with leg circulation problems have reported good results from taking ginkgo biloba as well.

Ginkgo extract has been used in Chinese medicine for over 5,000 years. It has been used as an antidote for aging, as well as for various spiritual uses. The ginkgo extract seems to enhance the function of neurotransmitters in our brain, as well as improve small vessel circulation, all of which help to enhance our memory.

Double blind studies of elderly individuals who were given 320 or 600 mg of ginkgo biloba extract had significant improvement in information processing. Other studies in which 120 mg of ginkgo were given per day showed improvement in cognitive function up to twenty-four weeks after having been given the herb.

Even patients suffering from senile macular degeneration had improvement in long distance vision acuity after getting ginkgo biloba.

I believe one of the greatest effects of ginkgo is its ability to improve circulation in very small capillaries, which is essential to feeding blood to the tiniest crevices of your brain, allowing greater connections to be made between various nerve pathways. In an earlier chapter, I stated that the more connectors you have, the greater will be your ability to make connections. Well, these connectors and connections are totally dependent on the circulation to that region. The more circulation you have in the smallest capillaries, the greater will be your ability to make these connections, and your memory will improve significantly.

Ginkgo appears to decrease the small capillary clotting, therefore increasing your circulation to these small blood vessels.

The heart can also be positively affected by ginkgo biloba by opening up its small collateral circulation when there is blockage in major blood vessels. Even arthritis patients and patients suffering from hepatitis, ringing in the ears, and Parkinson's disease have benefited from ginkgo extract.

Also, patients suffering from peripheral vision deficits as they get older seem to benefit from ginkgo by the increased circulation to the back of their eyes. Even diabetics suffering from diabetic retinopathy improved with the administration of ginkgo.

As you can see, based upon the history of the tree, which has been around for 200 million years, with each tree living up to 4000 years, we have a pretty good substance here that has a great chance of increasing longevity.

Ginkgo can be given in any condition where circulation has been a major impediment, and has led to stroke, brain disorders, memory problems, heart problems, and even neuropathy (where small nerve endings die away because of decreased capillary circulation).

As I see it, ginkgo biloba works similarly to chelation therapy in increasing your circulation. The only difference is that chelation therapy removes toxic metals from your body at the same time.

Taking ginkgo biloba may also increase the blood flow to the small blood vessels in your calves and thereby increase your ability to exercise and get the cardiovascular benefits of the anti-aging program.

If your impotency is caused by circulatory problems, ginkgo biloba may also have a beneficial effect in achieving and maintaining erections, along with vitamin E and chelation therapy.

Ginkgo also works as a potent antioxidant, preventing free radicals from destroying your cells, thus reducing the aging process itself. Ginkgo, therefore, should be an important component in the anti-aging regimen for brain health, along with constant mental stimulation to keep new neurons sprouting and making new connections. As long as these new neurons and dendrites have good circulation, along with adequate mental challenge, your mind should be as clear in old age as it was in youth. Ginkgo biloba is a very important component in keeping the mind sharp.

The usual dosage is 150 to 240 mg of 24% standardized extract of ginkgo biloba derived from the leaf itself. The 24% refers to the flavone glycoside component of the ginkgo. You want a standardized product which is measured against a laboratory reference, thereby identifying the exact amount you are getting.

It generally takes several months to get the beneficial effects of the ginkgo herb, so be patient and give it time. Just as with any other nutrient, it takes the body time to assimilate it into its biochemistry and to allow the beneficial effects to occur.

Other Free Radical Protective Supplements/Daily Doses of Important Supplements

We talked about vitamins A, C, E, and beta-carotene. We discussed Coenzyme Q10, selenium and the B vitamins. Now you may also consider ascorbyl palmitate, which is a fat-soluble form of vitamin C, as a supplement, along with zinc, manganese, and copper, which offer free radical production. Bioflavonoids are a very important group and work synergistically with vitamin C. They include rutin, hesperidin, quercetin, and Pycnogenol, along with ginkgo, which is a bioflavonoid.

Certain amino acids, such as glutamine, glutathione, methionine, cystine, and N-acetyl cysteine also offer free radical protection.

There is a group of potent bioflavonoid compounds called OPCs (Oligomeric Proanthocyanidins). This group of plant metabolite antioxidant compounds are present in hawthorn, nuts, apples, cinnamon, blueberry, bilberry, as well as grape seed extract, green tea, cranberries, red grape skins, red wines, lemon tree bark, peanut skins, the peels of oranges and Pycnogenol, which is derived from pine bark.

OPC compounds are very potent free radical scavengers and work synergistically with vitamin E and C. These compounds have also shown to be antibacterial, antiviral, anti-inflammatory, vasodilators and anti-allergic. You may want to include them in your anti-aging program.

Green tea, a popular beverage in China and Japan, has been shown to be effective on stomach cancers as well as esophageal cancers in women, and had protective effects in both male and female smokers. It is also useful against heart disease, which is a common problem in aging. Green tea was also shown to decrease total serum cholesterol in a Japanese study.

Dosage Ranges of Various Supplements Prescribed by Integrative Medicine Physicians

(Mostly derived from the
Longevity Medicine Supplement lectures at the ACAM anti-aging
courses and other sources.)

As mentioned previously, talk with a healthcare professional before beginning any supplementation regimen as they potentially can significantly interact with prescription medications as well as with each other. It is advisable that the higher dosages be taken only under supervision of a physician familiar with the nutrient.

Vitamin A: 10,000 to 50,000 IU (international units). You need to be cautious when pregnant if you take more than 10,000 IU, or 3,000 micrograms/d, since birth defects may occur. As well, liver damage can arise in some people. (One microgram equals 3.33 IU.)

Carotenoids: 15,000 to 50,000 IU, preferably mixed carotenoids rather than beta-carotene alone.

Vitamin B1(Thiamine): 50 to 500 mg.

Vitamin B2 (Riboflavin): 50 to 500 mg.

Vitamin B3 (Niacin, Niacinamide, or Inositol Hexaniacinate): 50 to 3000 mg.

Vitamin B5: (Pantothenic acid or calcium pantothenate): 100 to 2000 mg. Incidentally, 900 mg pantethene in a coenzyme form of pantothenate appears to lower cholesterol.

Vitamin B6 (Pyridoxine): 50 to 300 mg daily. Caution, in high dosages of 500 to 6,000 mg you may get neuropathy, so the dosage needs to be monitored.

Vitamin B12 (Cyanocobalamine): 100 to 1000 mcg daily. People often take the higher dosage in intramuscular injections as hydroxycobalamin.

Folic acid: 800 to 80,000 mcg (80 mg). At 80 mg, it has been used for gout. While 5 mg is a common folic acid dosage, during pregnancy, 1 to 5 mg is used..

Vitamin C: 2 to 50 grams, either oral, intravenous, or in combination. That may sound like a high dosage. Some people take about 4-5 grams a day in a powdered form in juice. Others have used the high dosages successfully as an IV drip, especially in fighting fatal diseases. 1-2 grams in pill form is more common for general use.

Vitamin D: 200 to 400 IU, older people may need the higher dose.

Vitamin E: 400 to 3,000 IU, preferably in a mixed state, as previously mentioned, of alpha, beta, delta, and gamma. It has to be a natural form of vitamin E. Synthetic vitamin E, d-l-Alpha tocopherol generally should not exceed 800 IU. The natural form has been taken at the higher dosages.

Coenzyme Q10: 100 to 400 mg; or occasionally higher, up to 600 mg. It is taken in oil-based or lecithin chewable forms.

Magnesium: 500 to 1,000 mg. Magnesium has a calming effect on muscles, agitation and anxiety. It helps with constipation and is often used as a natural sleep aid.

Calcium: 500 to 1,000 mg.

Chromium: 200 to 1,200 mcg. The higher dosages are used in diabetes treatment.

Selenium: 200 to 1,000 mcg. Again, the higher dosages are sometimes used in treating certain diseases. .

Zinc: 15 to 80 mg. It is used in combination of 10:1 or 15:1 with copper.

Copper: 2 to 5 mg.

Manganese: 10 to 20 mg.

L-glutamine: 2 to 8 grams. (It can be absorbed through the blood brain barrier.) It is also given in combination with ginkgo biloba for memory.

L-carnitine: 500 to 2,000 mg.

Taurine: 1,000 to 3,000 mg. Taurine has been found to be beneficial in maintaining retinal function and it is sometimes added to an intravenous chelation drip for people with macular degeneration. Taurine has also been used experimentally on rabbits with induced congestive heart failure and has been found to be beneficial.

Mixed Bioflavonoids: 1,000 to 4,000 mg

Quercetin: 800 to 1,600 mg. Quercetin is used as an anti-inflammatory and an anti-allergy agent and appears to inhibit histamine release which decreases inflammation.

Ginkgo Biloba: 120 to 240 mg at 24% standardized extract, as explained previously.

Proanthocyanidins OPC: 50 to 200 mg, usually as a grape seed extract or pine bark extract, and sometimes a mixture of both with red wine extract, citrus peel extract or bilberry extract. Many people feel Pycnogenol may be an even more potent antioxidant than vitamins E and C.

Silymarin extract (milk thistle): 150 to 600 mg of 80% standardized extract. This is obtained from the seed shell of the milk thistle, which contains powerful bioflavonoid-like chemicals, used to protect the liver and rebuild damaged cells, such as in hepatitis, cirrhosis, and jaundice. Alpha Lipoic Acid, Selenium and Silymarin have been used successfully for Hepatitis C.

Echinacea: 250 to 1,000 mg of mixed standardized extract. Echinacea has been used as a powerful natural antibiotic by many people.

Garlic: 500 to 2,000 mg of deodorized powder. I personally prefer natural garlic, crushed.

Saw palmetto: 320 to 640 mg of standardized extract. Saw palmetto has been used effectively for prostatic hypertrophy.

Bilberry: 100 to 300 mg of 15% to 25% standardized anthocyanosides content. Bilberry has been shown to have vaso-protective and anti-edema effects in animal trials (protects blood vessels and swelling). It has also been shown to reduce ischemia (lack of blood supply) damage.

Melatonin: 0.5 to 6 mg at bedtime. Melatonin is a very important hormone that has been used for insomnia and jet lag. The most important part of melatonin is that it is a potent antioxidant and protects against free radical damage.

This is only a partial list of vitamins, minerals, and supplements. These are some of the cMc multivitamin and mineral supplements I used in my chelation practice.

At the *happylifehealthyaging.com* web site we will have vitamin options available for purchase as well as special boutique vitamin combinations.

cMc Multi-Vitamin, Mineral, Trace Element Supplements

(These were the pill supplement ingredients we used in our practice – dosages are per serving)

Vitamin A (Palmitate)	10,000 I.U.
Vitamin A (Beta Carotene Vitamin A Activity)	10,000 I.U.
Vitamin C (L-Ascorbic Acid Corn Free)	1,200 mg
Vitamin D-3 (Cholecalciferol)	200 I.U.
Vitamin E (d-Alpha Tocopheryl Succinate)	400 I.U.
Vitamin B-1 (Thiamine Mononitrate)	100 mg
Vitamin B-2 (Riboflavin)	50 mg
Vitamin B-3 (Niacin)	50 mg
Vitamin B-3 (Niacinamide)	150 mg
Vitamin B-6 (Pyridoxine HCL)	25 mg
Folic Acid (Folacin)	800 mcg
Vitamin B-12 (In ion Exchange Resin)	150 mcg

Biotin	300 mcg
Pantothenic Acid (d-Calcium Pantothenate)	350 mg
Calcium (Citrate)	500 mg
Iodine (Kelp)	200 mcg
Magnesium (Ascorbate, Aspartate, Gluconate and Oxide)	500 mg
Zinc (Gluconate Aspartate)	25 mg
Selenium (Amino Acid Complex Selenemax)	200 mcg
Manganese (Gluconate Aspartate)	25 mg
Copper (Amino Acid Chelate)	2 mg
Chromium (Amino Acid Chelate)	200 mcg
Molybdenum (Amino Acid Chelate)	100 mcg
Potassium (Gluconate Aspartate)	99 mg
Boron (Aspartate-Citrate)	1000 mcg
Choline (Bitartrate)	100 mg
Citrus Bioflavonoids	150 mg
Inositol	100 mg
PABA (Para Amino Benzoic Acid)	100 mg
Vanadium (Amino Acid Chelate)	30 mcg

Stearic Acid, Microcrystalline Cellulose, Croscarmellose Sodium, Hydroxypropyl Cellulose, Magnesium Stearate, Silicon Dioxide, Ethylcellulose and Sodium Lauryl Sulfate.

Once again, supervision by a knowledgeable physician is highly recommended when taking supplements. With such a wide variety, it is easy to become carried away and take hundreds of pills a day. For most people, the basic list of C, E, B-complex, selenium, along with good multivitamins and trace minerals, should be adequate for antioxidant protection. Some people often want to add OPCs to the supplement list due to their potent antioxidant effects. The list of supplement dosages is meant only as a reference point for you while checking the content of your own multivitamin and mineral supplements. This list gives you a reference to go by in evaluating the potency of the supplements you are taking.

As you can see from this extensive list, supplements can become quite confusing. A healthy diet with colored fruits and vegetables of five servings a day will give you many of the essential minerals and vitamins you need. However, due to the free radical damage that is occurring through all the pollutants in our environment, extra supplements may be needed as insurance, and the potent antioxidants, vitamins and minerals, as described in this chapter, are a good way to start protecting yourself from oxidative stress and micronutrient depletion.

Take a clue from nature… Oxford University researchers observed chimpanzees in the Uganda Budongo Forest eating kaolinite clay to detoxify and boost their mineral content. The long term study, published in PLoS ONE in 2015, described how the mineral source for the chimps (raffia palm leaves) had diminished, so they started supplementing their diet with clay. Do the chimps know something that we don't?

Now for the bad news:

When I reviewed new studies of literature on vitamins and minerals, I kept on seeing one publication that was consistently being mentioned by several journals. The A4M (*American Academy for Anti-Aging Medicine*) web site had an article revealing proof of the efficacy of vitamins. The article first appeared in the prestigious journal *Nutrition*, in 2001, and was authored by a famous doctor (name omitted for legal reasons) at Memorial University in St Johns, Newfoundland, Canada. I was so impressed by the results that I planned a visit to see this renowned researcher at his lab, to review the data and talk to his research assistants about other benefits they noticed but did not publish. This man had been a renowned immunologist and nutrition researcher for 30 years, having published dozens of publications on infant formulas, nutrition and immunology.

His publication indicated that in people 65 years of age or older, a combination of supplements consisting of 18 vitamins and minerals increased immunity, increased short term memory, increased attention span, and decreased the rate of infection by as much as 50%. It also indicated that one US Dollar in supplements would save 28 dollars in health care by preventing or delaying illness and functional deficits. When I first read this, I obviously became very excited because it would show the value of vitamins and minerals in a standardized epidemiologic study.

Curious about his results, I researched his findings as much as I could. As it turned out, I was not the only one that became skeptical of his experiment; other scientists also questioned the validity of his results and asked to see the raw data. The data could not be found. You know the saying: "If it sounds too good to be true, it is too good to be true." I will spare you all the details. The researcher ended up resigning (retiring) from the University and the journal "Nutrition" retracted the publication in 2005. The Canadian Broadcasting Corporation (CBC) did a thorough investigation of the researcher, his data, and alleged research. Their findings can be found on the internet.

Subsequently, however, the *Annals of Internal Medicine* did do an extensive review of vitamin studies and published their findings on April 3, 2013. They found some benefit, but, essentially, indicated that eating the proper foods is just as beneficial and you may just be wasting your money on vitamins.

The NCCIH (National Center for Complementary and Integrative Health), a division of NIH (National Institutes of Health), reviewed several recent trials using antioxidant supplements for specific diseases. Most trials showed no disease-specific effects by the supplements tested. It was hypothesized that vegetables and fruits had additional components that were not in the supplements tested.

In the Selenium and Vitamin E Prostate Cancer Prevention Trial (SELECT), using more than 35,000 men aged 50 or older, it was found that selenium and vitamin E supplements, taken either alone or together, did not prevent prostate cancer. A 2011 updated analysis concluded that Vitamin E alone increased occurrence of prostate cancer by 17 percent as opposed to a placebo, but Vitamin E plus selenium showed no increase of prostate cancer.

While Macular Degeneration occurs in older individuals and leads to central vision loss, some 2 million US retirees experience severe vision loss. The cause of this disease is unknown. It is only second to cataracts in causing severe vision impairment. If you are over 70 yrs old, your chances of getting this disease start increasing rapidly. So what can you do? Reduce your correlated risk factors such as smoking, or having high blood pressure, and increase leafy green vegetables, anti-oxidants and carrots. Estrogen supplementation in post-menopausal women seems to reduce the risk of advanced wet macular degeneration.

Ophthalmologists have lasered wet macular degeneration vessels to stop their progression; unfortunately, this lasering technique leads to some loss of vision at the laser target sites. Various chemotherapy drugs have been tried in order to stop the leakage of the blood vessels inside the eye. In 2001 and 2013, research on Age Related Eye Disease Studies (AREDS), as sponsored by the National Eye Institute and various NIH divisions, was released. The studies found that the most beneficial treatment to prevent progression of dry macular degeneration towards the bad wet macular degeneration was the use of vitamins. The first study found that using Vitamins C (500mg), E (400IU), A (beta carotene, 15 mg), Zinc (Zn, 80mg) and Copper (cuprous oxide, 2mg) had beneficial effects. In the 2013 follow-up study they recommended adding Omega 3 fatty acids (DHA, EPA) found in fish. They also recommended Lutein (10mg) and Xeaxanthin which are micronutrients found in the human macula and can be obtained through leafy green vegetables and eggs.

Now for the big news: The study found a 25% reduction in the risk of progression from dry macular degeneration to the bad wet macular degeneration by supplementing your diet with these antioxidant nutrients. The use of antioxidant supplements alone reduced the risk by about 17 percent. In the same study, however, it was found that antioxidants did not help to prevent cataracts or slow their progression. Macular Degeneration is a terrible disease and these antioxidant findings may help improve many people's vision.

Studies such as these justify the use of vitamins for me. The *Annals of Internal Medicine* studies had people taking a very low dose of coated multivitamins for prevention use. The rebuttals that I have read questioned the quality of the vitamins, the coatings, and colorings used. The quality, bioavailability, and absorbability of vitamins in their natural co-factor form seem to be very important in the body's usage of them. Green leafy vegetables have all the co- factors needed for absorption. These co-factors should also be present in high quality supplements for optimal health results.

One more thing regarding vitamins: Spina Bifida is a birth defect in which the protective structure around spinal cord does not close completely and can cause death or various degrees of paralysis. The incidence of spina bifida used to be 1/1000 live births. Since the advent of Folic Acid supplementation, the incidence has decreased to 1/2000 – 3000 live births.

If we get all the vitamins we need through food, why has the incidence of this terrible birth defect improved with the use of this B vitamin? The reason is that our artificially engineered food does not contain enough of this needed vitamin to help prevent this defect.

Personally, I see no need to change my opinions about vitamins, minerals and trace nutrients, for the time being. In the summer of 2015, at the medical research department of Memorial University in Newfoundland, I stumbled on posters taped to the wall of the hallway. The posters were of recent research done at the University. One poster was titled: "Higher Dietary Magnesium Intake is Associated with Reduced Insulin Resistance in the Newfoundland Population." Now this is a big deal for those that are pre-diabetic. Data like this exists all over the place. Hippocrates, the father of medicine stated "Let food be thy medicine and medicine be thy food." Vitamins are elements of food. Our food's nutritional content is being diminished. In order to have the finest building blocks for your cells to replicate and perform optimally, we need the adequate nutrients for the cells to do their job. Vitamin and mineral supplementation augments what we eat. Many of us do not eat enough of the proper food mix to give us all the vitamins and minerals we need. Moreover, as we age, our gut may not absorb the vitamins and minerals adequately, so boosting their supply is probably a good idea and having a good mix of gut flora is beneficial as well. The decision is up to you. Antioxidants are key ingredients in fighting our modern degenerative diseases. The latest research supports what I published 15 years ago in *7 Secrets of Anti-Aging*.

We are exposed to free radicals daily. Sources of free radicals include cigarette smoke, air pollution, and even sunlight. Free radicals can cause "oxidative stress," and oxidative stress can cause cell damage. Oxidative stress is thought to play a role in a variety of diseases including cancer, cardiovascular diseases, diabetes, Alzheimer's disease, Parkinson's disease, eye diseases such as cataracts, as well as age-related macular degeneration and skin damage causing age spots and skin cancer.

In laboratory experiments on animals, antioxidants have been shown to counteract the oxidative stress effect. However, there is debate on whether consuming large amounts of antioxidants in supplements actually benefits health, and whether excessive quantities of certain antioxidants such as vitamin E or beta carotene may be harmful. The best sources of antioxidants are fruits and vegetables. However, with the nutrient depletion of these sources, supplementation may be wise (if not taken in excess quantities), especially of the fat soluble vitamins.

The vitamins that are manufactured from natural sources with all the co-factors that exist in fruits and vegetables may be the wisest choice to take. A high quality vitamin with co-factors found in nature, is expensive to produce and costs more than the cheap mass-produced vitamins you can find anywhere. Your body is the most valuable thing that you own, doesn't it make sense to give it the highest quality nutrients available? We will have a list of quality supplements, from a variety of companies, on our web site.

There are various other nutrients used for health, such as saw palmetto, a supplement that many use for benign prostatic hypertrophy and frequent urination. This book focuses on optimizing your chances for healthy aging rather than on healing specific conditions. Other nutrients will be discussed on our web site without making specific health claims. Specific health claims can only be made by drug companies after spending millions of dollars on double-blind placebo controlled studies for individual illnesses.

Individually, it is hard to keep up with all the new research on longevity and anti-aging. To help, you can periodically log on to the *happylifehealthyaging.com* web site to see what we have found.

CHAPTER 7

Hormone Replacements

It's a beautiful Monday morning. The sun is glistening over the ocean. The humpback whales are breaking through the water for a few moments after feeding on herring and krill before diving back towards the ocean floor. The air is filled with a cool, salty, breeze. What a gorgeous spot to re-write this chapter on hormones at beautiful Cape Spear, Newfoundland, Canada. The Cape Spear lighthouse, just south of St John's, sits on a mountainous cliff and is the easternmost point of Continental America. The beauty of nature surrounds me as I delve into the world of hormones, an essential element to our existence and enjoyment of life.

Many years ago, my twelve-and-a-half-year-old daughter told me, "Daddy, you know, I just feel so angry inside and so yuck. I have no reason for it; I just feel that way. Nothing happened in the day that made me angry, or don't have a reason to be mad at anyone. It's just the way I feel."

I sat back and said to myself, that's hormones. Young bucks on a Saturday night, hot to trot, getting all dolled up, waxing their cars, slicking their hair, putting on the newest duds just so they can ride up and down the road in a convertible with their buddies, looking at all the girls, whistling at them, and acting silly among themselves. That's hormones, too.

Hormones are little tiny chemical messengers that are secreted into our blood stream and go to specific target organs and influence them to act in a certain way. It could be for sexual stimulation/arousal. It could be for growth of tissues, such as muscles. It may also be for maintenance and healing, or repair of tissues. The word hormone comes from the Greek "hormaein" meaning to spur on, to edge on, or to set in motion. A good description, isn't it? Facilitation is another word you can use for it.

Why do you think eunuchs were the ones that guarded the harems? Was it because those big burly guys were more trustworthy than the rest of the soldiers the Sultan had, or was it because their testicles had been removed at an early age and they had no hormones?

Eunuchs were not sexually aroused by beautiful young women with voluptuous bodies. They weren't aroused because they had no male hormones.

What about those young boys with great singing voices in the middle ages? Some people thought those voices needed to be preserved. To make sure a boy's voice didn't change to a man's voice as his hormone levels kicked in, his testicles were amputated before he reached puberty.

The Castrati were the singing rock stars of Europe during the 1700s and early 1800s. Women would swoon over them because of their beautiful high-pitched voices.

In the Forbidden City, in China, I was told that Eunuchs were the only males allowed (other than the emperors and their direct families) because they could be trusted with the women living there.

You see, a lot of characteristics we have are hormone-induced. You may notice that as young children go through adolescence they start developing specific body features, such as curves for girls, and lean, tough muscles for boys. All these secondary sexual characteristics are hormone-induced, just as our growth itself is hormone-induced.

However, having too much growth hormone makes people grow very large and tall and they can acquire large bones; while with too little, or no growth hormone, people stay very, very short.

Hormones are produced through glands, which are part of the system called the endocrine system. Hormone levels change over time. Unfortunately, as we get older, there are fewer hormones being produced.

Scientifically, taking evolution as a guide, there is very strong evidence implicating the endocrine system as a major regulator of aging and life span. It controls many aspects of our existence from mood, sexual reproduction, and growth, to metabolism and stress resistance.

Some of the hormones that decrease with age are testosterone, estrogen, androgens, aldosterone, DHEA, growth hormone, thyroid hormone, and even insulin (which is the hormone diabetics take to make sure they get adequate blood sugar going into their muscles).

So what do hormones have to do with longevity? Well, as I just mentioned, vital hormones decrease with age. If we can somehow increase these hormones to the level of when we were younger, we can, to a certain extent, reverse the detrimental changes that occur due to their inevitable depletion.

What we want to do is put ourselves into a physiological state similar to when we were 40years old, and have the same level of hormones we had then.

Influencing a host of processes in our bodies, hormones can then optimize our energy levels, muscles, cardiac function, and the fight/flight mechanism. These are influenced by powerful hormones such as cortisol, adrenaline, or epinephrine (the charging tiger inside us), and can affect sexual stamina, arousal, and performance to the level of a younger person.

The endocrine system is a finely tuned one. Like a Tango, all of the hormones dance together, and they have to be perfectly in step with one another. Small changes can make big differences. The basic rule: The more natural the hormone, the better the results. Synthetic hormones have produced some tragedies with their use.

Unnatural estrogens and progesterones have increased the cancer level of some women and caused them to die early of uterine or ovarian cancers. An improper hormone ratio may also produce unwanted consequences.

Now, speaking of hormone imbalance, how about the crop spraying of pesticides that we continuously absorb, and that interfere with our endocrine system?

Or, how about the hormones given to chicken and beef to accelerate their growth so that they can then be sold and processed more rapidly for greater profit? How about the hormones and medications in ground water?

We absorb these hormones day in and day out without even realizing it, and, more than likely, are altering our endocrine system more and more. Indiscriminate use of hormones can, potentially, be very, very dangerous.

Whenever a drug company tries to mimic nature, be cautious. Read about synthetic hormones, especially their side effects or adverse reactions in the Physicians Desk Reference manual. Unless a hormone is exactly like the one we naturally produce, it cannot participate in the dance of the hormones. (Some genetically engineered hormones, however, can be identical.)

Synthetic hormones are not natural. The body is not accustomed to using them. However, they mimic our natural hormones enough so that they can occupy spaces in our cells called receptors, yet they don't function quite as well.

Because synthetic hormones occupy these receptors, natural hormones cannot get in since "the keyholes" are full. It's like somebody making a copy of a key for a lock. However, it isn't exactly right. You put it into the keyhole and it fits, but it doesn't open the lock, or it sticks and is difficult, and you have to jog it around to make the lock open.

Well, that's what a synthetic hormone is. It doesn't quite work right. And, because it doesn't work right, it creates a host of complications which can be deadly to our system.

So, a word of caution about synthetic hormones:
READ THE LIST OF SIDE EFFECTS.
The body is finely tuned. You do not want to throw it out of balance to the point where it becomes fatal.

Now, the good news. Among the myriad hormones in our endocrine system, some influence our life span; therefore, replacing them as they decline makes some sense.

However, whenever you are tweaking the finely tuned endocrine system, you have to be careful. The hormones are the messengers telling the other parts of your body what to do. If you are getting wrong messages, wrong things are going to happen.

Whenever doctors prescribe hormonal changes, they start with low dosages and go slowly and cautiously.

Human Growth Hormone (HGH)

What if I told you that a published study reported that in six months they found:

* increased memory retention
* higher energy level
* enhanced sexual performance
* an 8.8% increase in muscle mass without exercise

* stronger bones
* faster wound healing
* hair regrowth
* improved sleep
* younger, tighter, thicker skin with removal of wrinkles
* elimination of cellulite
* sharper, clearer vision
* improved mood
* improved cholesterol profile with higher levels of HDL and lower levels of LDL, the bad cholesterol
* lower blood pressure
* better immune function
* regrowth of liver, heart, kidneys, spleen, as well as other organs that shrink as we get older
* greater cardiac output/increased exercise performance
* better kidney function
* 14.4% loss of fat on the average, after six months without dieting. That's right. You lose fat; you do not have to do anything, just pop this pill.

All of this sounds wonderful doesn't it? Well, Dr. Daniel Rudman completed a study, which was published in 1990 in the *New England Journal of Medicine*. He was at the Medical College of Wisconsin in Milwaukee, studying 61 to 81-year-olds and giving them human growth hormone. Guess what he found: improvements in every category that I mentioned above.

All of his male subjects had low levels of human growth hormone in their blood. He divided them into two groups. One group, of twelve men, received human growth hormone (HGH) injections three times a week for six months; the other group received nothing. By the end of the study his findings proved to be astounding.

His conclusions were that all these changes in our body, such as increased fat, decreased bone density, loss of muscle mass, decreased sexual energy, etc., are due to the decrease of growth hormone as we age.

The men who were given growth hormone injections three times a week had a reversal of these age-related changes that made them, in effect, ten to twenty years younger in muscle composition, fat distribution, and bone strength. He also found that skin thickness increased by 7.1% and the lower back bones, known as the lumbar vertebrae, increased by 1.6% in density.

In my experience, I noticed that patients who had human growth hormone injections prescribed by other doctors appeared more youthful, more energetic, and leaner. Some were aggressive and determined, and somehow, sexier. A word of caution here. If one partner does this and the other does not, you are going to have a great mismatch in sexual energy, which could cause tremendous problems in your marriage.

I remember seeing before-and-after photos of a couple in swim suits who took growth hormone injections. The contrast between the photos was absolutely astounding. The "after" pictures seemed to have been taken ten to twenty years earlier.

The woman looked younger and more vibrant. Her overall curves were that of a younger person. She had less fat, more contours, and didn't have baggy, sagging skin. She looked a heck of a lot sexier than the before picture. The man lost the inner tube around his waist. He had much more muscle definition and a more vigorous appearance.

Both of them appeared much younger, all due to the hormone injections. This shows you how powerful this hormone is, as we are growing up, in tuning our bodies to peak performance.

Visible changes are slow to occur, and you generally have to wait six months to a year before you see anything happen. But the results I saw in this couple, as well as in other patients who have taken the hormone injections, were dramatic. The growth hormone effect, however, plateaus after a while.

This hormone is at its highest level when we are at a childbearing age, and need to be most attractive in order to attract the opposite sex to procreate. Also, we men have to be strong and able to defend our spouse and children in case of an attack. So, this hormone causes us to grow while at the same time allowing us to be strong and attractive with lots of energy, because energy is needed at this point in our lives.

However, when your family is fully grown and you are more secure, there's no more need for this growth hormone and the body starts reducing it. As it shuts down, all the characteristics that made us attractive, strong, and full of sexual and physical energy start waning because there isn't the need for them. Kind of sad, isn't it? Wouldn't it be nice to be at that peak performance until you die?

Well, everything has its price. HGH (human growth hormone) injections will cost you about $8,000 to $10,000 a year and you have to keep injecting yourself three times per week.

A word of caution, however. We do not know what the long-term consequences are of chronic HGH (human growth hormone) usage is.

Let me repeat that. We do not know what the long term consequences are of chronic human growth hormone usage.

Since growth hormone causes rapid growth, will it cause cancer to grow? Will there be a greater incidence of breast cancer, prostate cancer, or any other type of cancer because it stimulates growth? The answers are not in yet. However, in observing acromegalics (people who have had very high levels of HGH throughout their lives), it appears that they have fairly stable existences, but, on average, die 10 years younger mostly due to cardiovascular complications. They also have problems such as carpal tunnel syndrome due to enlarged hands. Conversely, with growth hormone replacement you are not getting the excessively high levels of growth hormone that acromegalics have, you are just aiming to reach the level of a younger person.

I read about an eight-foot man who had excess growth hormone. His parents sent him to the circus to make a living. Unfortunately he ended up dying in his early twenties due to the excess of growth hormones in his body.

The FDA is, appropriately, taking a cautionary approach towards HGH replacement. Initially it was approved for children who had growth deficiencies. Recently, the FDA approved HGH for certain conditions resulting in HGH deficiency. The word deficiency is subject to interpretation.

If you are old and have low levels of HGH, are you deficient in HGH? Who makes that decision? Generally people who are getting HGH get their IGF-1 (insulin growth factor 1) levels checked periodically, which are indicators of HGH in your body as HGH is very difficult to measure. It is pulsatile and not very constant in your blood stream. IGF levels are much more level and easier to measure, and are an indicator of your HGH level. Anyway, these people get their IGF-1 levels measured periodically and try to maintain levels of a 30-year-old.

There is another way to take HGH. That is through HGH stimulators, called secretagogues. They stimulate our own anterior pituitary gland to produce more HGH. They are probably most effective for people in the 40 to 60 year-old range and include the amino acids arginine, ornithine, glutamine, and lysine. Based upon clinical observations, and reports from other physicians that I have talked to, the injectable form of HGH is probably better for people older than 60years old; and, the secretagogues, which would stimulate the anterior pituitary gland to produce its own growth hormone, would probably be better for the 40 to 60year-old group because there is still adequate growth hormone that can be released from the pituitary itself if stimulated. Once again, any attempt to alter your growth hormone level should be supervised by a licensed physician. This area in medicine is very controversial.

A new product is also being tested which is a transdermal growth hormone-releasing-factor. This releasing factor stimulates your pituitary gland to release growth hormone. It's easy to use; simply rub it over your hands and your skin will absorb it.

Some of you may be on a budget and can't just fork out $10,000 a year for these injections in order to look younger, be more physically vigorous, have less fat, and have your organs regrow. You may be asking, "Is there any other way I can increase my growth hormone level?" Well, yes, there is. And it's something that involves effort on your part. Yucky effort—but you don't want to make an effort, do you? You want to take that magic pill and grow young. Well, this is, I think, probably a much better way to get growth hormone: Physical Activity.

Physical activity, especially aerobic exercise, such as the Lenhart Physical Activity Anti-Aging Program that I mentioned several chapters ago, stimulates the release of HGH to the blood stream. Even if you are sedentary and suddenly become physically active, you have bursts of HGH released to your blood stream allowing you to feel younger in every way.

Remember the story about my neighbor who was on his death bed when he was seventy-four, then he became physically active and started walking twice a day? His pace became faster and faster. He became more vigorous. At eighty-four he was physically younger than he was at seventy-two. He looked younger and his muscles were younger. Why? Because, through his physical activity, he stimulates HGH release, which decreases body fat, increases muscle tone, increases organ size, and gives him more spunk and energy.

Yes, ladies and gentleman, physical activity is the poor man's growth hormone-stimulating-factor, and probably the safest.

The best thing is that you are doing it naturally. However, for those of you who are searching for ways other than physical activity, you can look at our Web site: *happylifehealthyaging.com.*

Some people are also using homeopathic doses of growth hormone, along with the secretagogues, and getting some positive results. You may also get a better effect with the secretagogues if you detoxify, or clean yourself out. You see, there is a theory that the hypothalamus gets plugged up with heavy metals and other toxins and is unable to stimulate the anterior pituitary in order to release growth hormone. If you detoxify yourself and your hypothalamus works better, it can stimulate the anterior pituitary so that you get more growth hormone release. It goes back to the entire concept of this book, that all of the Longevity Secrets are equally important.

Now for the bad news: Since the first edition of this book was published 15 years ago, more research has been completed on growth hormone. This newer research validates my cautious approach in the first edition of this book.

In recently published research papers on rodents, a deficiency of growth hormone, or nonfunctioning growth hormone receptors, has resulted in life extension. The deficiency itself may delay aging in rodents by enhancing antioxidative defenses, increase insulin sensitivity and increase stress resistance. Mice lacking growth hormone were considerably smaller. Researchers found that larger animals lived shorter lives. Growth hormone is considered diabetogenic by opposing the action of insulin. Humans, and mice, with high levels of Growth Hormone had increased insulin, were hyperglycemic, (high blood sugar), or were insulin resistant, and half of the humans became diabetic with blood vessel complications. This is not a good thing. Mice that were deficient in growth hormone had lower blood sugar, lower circulating insulin and increased insulin sensitivity. Significantly, this means that they could process the sugar more easily and therefore did not need as much in their blood. Unfortunately, they were also less fertile. That is why in the Rudman Growth Hormone study, the sexual characteristics in people were enhanced with supplemental growth hormone usage. You can't have it all.

By the way, insulin resistance increases with increased belly fat (making you more prone to diabetes) and decreases with abdominal fat loss. This is why the doctor at my hospital that went on the intermittent fast diet was able to control his diabetes, as well as his high blood pressure, without having to take medication.

So what do we have in this maze of confusing data? Growth Hormone is good and bad. There is a reason that it decreases with age and is high in our early fertile years. This is a field that is filled with risk, and you need to weigh the benefits and disadvantages with your doctor.

Melatonin

Have you ever wondered how birds find their way at night when migrating from Canada to Florida or South America? How do they navigate? How do they know when to start their migratory cycles? Is there a sign in the sky that says, "Hey, it's time to get out of here and go to warmer weather"? Or, how about the need to migrate back north after basking in the warm, tropical sun in the winter, all of a sudden picking up roots and tracking back one to two-thousand miles? What's the signal that makes animals do that?

How about the breeding cycles of animals? Some of them magically appear out of nowhere at a particular location, at a certain stream, or a certain patch of grass, every year at about the same time and they go at it! They have whoopie, produce their young, raise them, and then take off not to be seen again for another year. How do these animals know when to complete these cycles? Did you ever wonder about that?

Well, all those magical powers animals possess seem to be regulated by a little gland called the pineal gland, which sits in the middle of the brain. (Years ago doctors thought this gland was archaic and useless.) As you will recall, these glands regulate and stimulate all kinds of functions in animals and humans by being chemical messengers. Well, the pineal gland simulates, in part, the navigational ability and reproducibility of animals. It's a little like an internal clock that has its own rhythms of night and day, seasons, and reproductive cycles.

The pineal gland in humans is pea-sized. It is really small, but it has a tremendous influence on how we do things. Some people are night people and are more productive at night. They think more clearly at night, and get more accomplished. Others are morning people. They awaken at 5:00 a.m. and their day is very productive early on. By 8:00 p.m. they're tired and want to sleep.

All that timing somehow seems to be connected to the pineal gland. It monitors the length of the day and change in seasons. It triggers the reproductive systems of seasonally breeding mammals. It also helps regulate other hormones in these mammals to trigger when to start breeding or, even, shed their hair.

Why do dogs and other furry animals shed their hair at certain times of the year even though they aren't consciously aware of the changing seasons? It's all hormonal and is regulated by the pineal gland sensing the amount of daylight.

The pineal gland secretes a very important hormone in humans called melatonin. There were a series of studies in Italy, on mice, that were given melatonin-enriched water and they ended up living longer and became more sexually active and vigorous. They also acquired a better immune system than the mice that did not have melatonin-enriched water. The significant factor with these mice was that they did not produce melatonin naturally, so it was a great stimulant for them and in turn helped enhance their life cycle.

When the same experiment was repeated in mice that produced melatonin naturally, the findings were not replicated. For a while, melatonin was touted as the miracle anti-aging hormone. But it didn't exactly pan out like that.

Melatonin did, however, enhance the immune system. It was shown to be a very potent antioxidant, which reduces cell damage produced by free radicals.

Melatonin promotes sleep and is used by many people to help them sleep. It also alleviates jet lag and resets your day/ night clock fairly rapidly from those transatlantic flights.

So, instead of taking two to three days getting used to the new time zone, you may consider taking melatonin the night before your trip, and the first night there, helping you to quickly adapt to the new time zone and be up and running.

The newest theories are revealing how melatonin may play an important role in longevity by decreasing the free radical damage in your neurons through its potent antioxidant effect as a free radical scavenger. We all know what free radicals do: free radicals slowly bombard our cells and destroy them or alter them so much that mutations occur, which lead to life-threatening diseases. So, if you can mop up these free radicals, such as with melatonin and other antioxidants, you get a greater chance of gaining normal cell function, fewer disease processes, and greater enhancement and prolongation of life.

A friend of mine takes melatonin whenever she cannot sleep. It knocks her out and she gets a great night's sleep. Melatonin works best at night when the hormone is normally released by the body.

However, light seems to turn off the beneficial effect of melatonin. People who sleep with a night light, or the television on, or anything like that, really do themselves a great disservice because they are not getting adequate amounts of melatonin.

Just as melatonin regulates the day and night cycle for us, the migratory and reproductive cycles in birds and animals, and many other cycles you can think of, it may in fact be regulating your life cycle as well. Although not totally proven, there are strong indications that melatonin influences stages of your life, telling you when to start a new chapter of life.

What it is doing is setting your aging clock, kind of like an hour glass. When the sand runs out, it's time for you to go. It is a timing process. Melatonin may, in fact, be setting the pace at which you age. As it gradually decreases with age, there is less stimulation to your other hormones and you gradually wind down.

Well, let's see what else melatonin does. I heard a very interesting lecture by Russell J. Reiter, Ph.D., otherwise known as Mr. Melatonin, on the topic of melatonin, aging, and age-related neurodegenerative diseases. He is the foremost researcher on the topic of melatonin, and he is in the Department of Cellular and Structural Biology at the University of Texas Health Science Center, San Antonio. He has made it his life's work to study this one little hormone. It was a stimulating lecture for me because I did not realize all the other effects melatonin had on our bodies.

What did he and other researchers find? They've found that melatonin is a very potent free radical scavenger. We've known that since 1991.

Other studies have found that melatonin was roughly five times more effective as a scavenger destroying free radicals than another potent hydroxyl radical scavenger, known at glutathione.

Simply put, this stuff is darn potent in reducing and mopping up those free radicals. Better yet, melatonin works synergistically (works together in unison) to provide antioxidant protection with other free radical scavengers.

Not only that, it reduces free radical generation. That's even better. If fewer free radicals are produced, you'll have less damage occurring. And, guess what? By its synergetic action it helps recycle glutathione, another potent antioxidant now starting to be used in treating Parkinson's disease by decreasing symptomatology. Pretty interesting stuff.

The more we learn about free radical damage of our cells, the more we learn about chronic degenerative conditions that cause us to age prematurely. As we age, our cell membranes become progressively more rigid, in other words become more brittle, which interferes with the passage of all types of nutrients such as solutes (dissolved nutrients) across the cell membranes. This, in turn, alters something known as receptor processes, which we need for optimum cell function.

Those are a lot of fancy words to say we shrivel up. Well, melatonin prevents this shriveling process, such as lipid peroxidation, thereby keeping us softer. Just think of your skin. As it gets older, it gets brittle, thin, and breaks down easily. Well, melatonin sort of acts as a skin softener for your cells.

While melatonin is curtailing your lipid pro-oxidation, which is the brittleness of your membranes, it simultaneously is also reducing DNA damage. DNA is the basic molecular structure from which all cells are made. It is the genetic code that determines what every part of your body becomes and what you become. Well, that is damaged over time. Melatonin somehow curtails that damage by its antioxidant effect as well as its free-radical scavenging effect. Pretty neat stuff. For example, not only will your skin be softer, it will not be destroyed as readily. To me, that is a significant anti-aging effect.

Before we leave this topic, I would like to say that melatonin crosses the blood/brain barrier very easily. That means it can go across this barrier and be found in your central nervous system, that is, the brain, spinal cord, and so forth, minutes after it is administered. Therefore, it protects your brain from oxidative damage. That's the free radical damage associated with so many neurological conditions, such as Parkinson's disease and Alzheimer's disease. The brain does not produce its own melatonin, but it readily absorbs it as a protective agent.

The gut, also, produces its own melatonin as a protection against numerous toxins we ingest through our mouth, which in turn stimulate free radical production and causes us to age and develop diseases.

The potent antioxidant effect and mopping-up effect of melatonin assists in many major organs in our body - liver, muscles, brain, lungs, eye lenses, stomach, and kidneys, all of which are susceptible to free radical attacks. Melatonin has direct and indirect anti-oxidative actions on many toxic substances, which in turn protects our body from aging. That makes melatonin one of the more important longevity substances you can take.

Perhaps you can reset your biological clock through increased intake of melatonin and live longer and healthier while at the same time enjoying restful sleep.

Some may wonder, "How safe is this substance?" I did raise the question of the safety of growth hormone earlier, but melatonin is in a totally different league. It is very, very safe. When extremely high doses were given to mice, to find out at what level half of them would die, none of them died.

In humans, up to 6,000 mg were given without any major side effects and with only an occasional upset stomach or lightheadedness. That's the best thing about melatonin, it is extremely safe and ranks high on my list as one of the best anti-aging products you can take.

The dosage of melatonin most people take is approximately 1 ½ to 3 mg, although some people take up to 10 mg at night. I find that 3 mg is more than adequate for most people and will produce a very deep sleep while at the same time fighting free radicals that are constantly ravaging your body, especially in the brain and central nervous system. I am convinced that as time goes on, we will learn more and more about this wonderful hormone and its many beneficial effects.

According to the NCCIH web site:

Research is being completed on adding melatonin to standard cancer care in order to improve response rates, survival time, and quality of life.

Results from a few small studies (clinical trials) on people have led investigators to propose additional research on whether melatonin may help to improve mild cognitive impairment in patients with Alzheimer's disease.

Sleep is a very important factor with dementia patients, and getting a good night's sleep makes a big difference in how alert someone is.

Melatonin is also being studied for prevention of cell damage associated with amyotrophic lateral sclerosis (ALS, also known as Lou Gehrig's disease). An analysis of the research suggested that adding sustained-release melatonin (but not fast-release melatonin) to a high blood pressure management regime reduced elevated nighttime blood pressure.

DHEA (Dehydroepiandrosterone)

It's a beautiful day here in mid-February in central Florida, in the Tampa Bay region. I am anchored at a place called DeSoto Point, the same place where Hernando DeSoto landed looking for his fortune, and where legend has it that Ponce de Leon was looking for the Fountain of Youth. As a matter of fact, it is a national park. You can row a dinghy in, get a tour of the area, and watch a historic video about how DeSoto trekked through Florida looking for a fortune.

As I rowed in this morning, for a communal breakfast that we had with a group of other sailors, I was offered a ride in another dinghy. However, I told them I wanted to get some exercise and row in. The conversation proceeded to why I was alone on the boat instead of with my kids and family. I told them I was writing a book on anti-aging and I needed some peace and quiet to dictate this chapter. The first thing a gentleman said was, "Is it going to do me any good?" "Yes, of course it will." "Am I going to be able to understand it." he asked? I told him that this book has been written as simply as possible in order for him. and others who are not medically-oriented. to reap its benefits.

It doesn't do you any good to hear a bunch of scientific names that have absolutely no meaning to you other than gibberish. I'm making every effort possible to limit the information to the most promising supplements which I feel have potential longevity benefits. If you look at the hormones and all their precursors, you could end up with hundreds of individual hormones where each has a specific effect. However, taken together they work like a unified football team by trying to establish balance in your endocrine system and through that balance influence a host of biological processes throughout your body.

Believe it or not, the thing that starts it all is cholesterol. Although cholesterol may be thought of with a negative connotation it is essential for our hormone function. I have a sneaking suspicion that in the long term all these cholesterol-lowering drugs will have harmful effects on our hormonal balance. There is a reason why some people's cholesterol is elevated and that of others is not.

Yes, it is diet-related to a certain extent, but also the body may have certain needs that it compensates for by manufacturing greater levels of cholesterol. When you throw off your body's own regulatory mechanism, you're asking for trouble.

Yes, cholesterol can be bad for you if it is oxidized and sticks to your blood vessels. However, if it is in a balanced formula with other chemicals in your body, such as omega-3 fatty acids derived from fish oils, cholesterol in itself is safe. You only run into trouble when you add the pollutants, toxins, and free radicals. These factors oxidize the cholesterol, make it stick, and then a physical obstruction occurs. But most of that is a byproduct of our lifestyles, the foods we consume, and the pollutants we inhale or are exposed to.

Let's look at one of the main byproducts of cholesterol, which is pregnenolone, a precursor to DHEA. Pregnenolone is like the first link in a chain of reactions of steroid hormones, which eventually leads to creating over a hundred different hormones.

Some of the hormones you get are DHEA, progesterone, testosterone and cortisol, as well as estrone, estradiol, and estriol (which are the three basic estrogens). . Pregnenolone is important in the immune system, sleep patterns, wound healing, anti-inflammatory reactions, stress reduction, and feelings of well-being. It blocks the effect of cortisol, a detrimental steroid, which is produced at very high stress levels.

Pregnenolone also improves our memory and concentration, helps alleviate depression, and assists with inflammatory diseases, such as arthritis, and the associated joint swelling that accompanies it. People have even used the hormone for psoriasis, lupus, and other skin and connective disorders, such as scleroderma. Almost anything that causes an inflammatory response due to an overproduction of cortisol has been found to be ameliorated by pregnenolone. If you look at the chain of conversions that occur from cholesterol, you'll see that pregnenolone converts to DHEA, which in turn converts to other hormones, such as estrogen, progesterone, testosterone, and cortisol.

So, what you are doing by taking DHEA is affecting a slew of hormones that are beneficial to your body in protecting you from age-related diseases, such as atherosclerosis, diabetes, cancer, immune disorders, and stress-induced disorders. Some people are even taking it for chronic fatigue and depression because it is a feel-good hormone. With it, people can think better, handle stress better. One study showed improvement in self-reported physical and psychological well-being in post-menopausal women. Did you know that DHEA is the most abundant hormone in the body? That's why it is so darned important.

However, the bad news is that it decreases as we age at 2-4% per year. It peaks around age twenty. It is at half of its level at age forty. By the time you are sixty-five, DHEA is at about fifteen percent of its optimum levels. By the time you're eighty, only five percent of the normal amount is still there. It is a very important anti-aging hormone because it is the precursor in a whole series of cascading events that produce hormones and that are protective to our body's organ systems and reproductive systems.

In going to seminars given by DHEA experts at the American Academy for the Advancement of Medicine, where I was one of the instructors in the anti-aging course, I listened to experts talk about the experiments being done with this hormone and was amazed as to why the world of medicine had not jumped at this remarkable product much earlier. The problem, as I soon realized, was the same problem with many other naturally-occurring substances.

It cannot be patented. Big pharmaceutical companies will not invest hundreds of millions of dollars in a product that is natural. They would rather try to come up with synthetic products so that they can then make tremendous profits. Natural products are of no use to them because they can't be patented.

The problem with the synthetic products produced by the drug companies is that they're not exactly the same as the natural products that have developed over hundreds of millions of years.

When we start taking synthetic products, such as horse-urine derived estrogen or synthetic progesterone, we run into trouble.

Yes, these products can be patented, and are prescribed extensively by doctors, but what effect are they having on the bodies of post-menopausal females? Why are certain reproductive system cancers increasing with the females taking these products? I'll tell you why. We don't know what we are doing and nature does.

Whenever you take a hormone, try to take it in as natural a form as possible. If it is a bio-engineered product, make sure it is exactly molecule-to-molecule to that of a natural human product. Otherwise, you are potentially asking for trouble.

Since DHEA is a precursor to the reproductive hormones, it should be an important component in hormone replacement protocols of post-menopausal females, as well as males. Because production of DHEA declines with age, as do our other hormones, and since it is the precursor of other hormones, DHEA would be a wise choice in an anti-aging program. Think of it this way: If the hundreds of hormones are snowballs trying to hit specific targets, DHEA would be the snow from which the snowballs are made. Cholesterol would be the water that crystallizes into the snowflakes. Does that make sense to you? You're throwing the snowballs at specific targets. The more snow you have, the more snowballs you can throw.

DHEA is manufactured in the adrenal cortex, which is a little gland above your kidneys. For years I have warned patients not to burn out their adrenals by excessive stress, excessive caffeine consumption, or excessive sugar consumption because I knew that vital hormones were being produced by that gland, hormones that are necessary to our survival, longevity, and repair mechanisms. The adrenal cortex is responsible, through its hormone production, for things such as muscle strength, immune response, and our overall stress level and quality of life.

DHEA is also bio transformed into biologically active estrogens and androgens (male hormones) in our tissues. Estimates are that over 90% of estrogen in postmenopausal women and 30% of total male hormones are derived from this tissue conversion.

In studies where 50 mg of DHEA were given to older individuals with low DHEA levels, the people taking the DHEA had their levels restored to that of young adults within two weeks. After three months, they found an increased level of the male sex hormones with people having an increase in physical, as well as psychological, well-being and a change in sex drive.

In studies performed on Alzheimer's patients, guess what? Low levels of DHEA were found. DHEA is essential in maintaining brain/nerve functions. It increases the REM sleep, which is the important part of sleep that is involved in memory storage and gives us complete rest.

It assists us in memory retention, as well as in depression. DHEA has even improved memory in mice. Other studies have shown DHEA to be effective in reducing lupus flare-ups, as well as improving glucose intolerance, which leads to diabetes. There are even studies done on mice that show a decrease in body fat when fed DHEA.

By now you're probably wondering, how can this one hormone do all these things? Well, it doesn't. Remember the snowball effect?

It manufactures the snowballs that have all these beneficial effects by stimulating the production of hundreds of other hormones.

I found an interesting study done on calorically restricted monkeys, where the DHEA level was higher in the calorically restricted monkeys than the control group. That reinforces to me the value of caloric restriction as an important component of your longevity program.

People taking synthetic estrogens or progesterone have had increased cancer incidents because they are bombarding the body with only one type of hormone.

One benefit I see in taking DHEA is that it does not overload the hormone system with a specific hormone that may throw everything out of balance. Since DHEA is a precursor of the other hormones, it will manufacture the necessary hormones your body needs in appropriate proportions. That's why I think no studies (as far as I know) exist where cancers have been increased with DHEA because the body will only take as much as is needed.

Generally, doses of DHEA are between 25 and 2,500 mg per day. However, you have to be careful because DHEA is converted into other hormones, so people with prostate cancer, benign prostatic hypertrophy, or women with reproductive cancers need to consult their physicians before taking DHEA. At least, try to find a physician who is familiar with its usage. Although I cannot recall, and have not been able to find, studies that have shown negative effects of DHEA with these conditions, a word of caution is advisable.

Balance, I believe, is the key to any longevity program. As in Shangri-La, the people were happy because of moderation and balance in their life. Everything outlined in this book is designed to give you a balanced approach towards healthy longevity. I tried to combine all aspects of anti-aging, as far as I am aware, towards optemising your life's extension and quality.

DHEA is an important hormone to take in your anti-aging program, but, with your doctor's help, you have to take the right amounts. Studies where people have taken 10 mg of DHEA showed no increase of wellbeing. However, larger dosages have had significant effects, including feeling better overall, increased blood levels of insulin growth factor, and enhancement of the immune function. So, you have to take the right dose.

How do you know you're taking the right amount of DHEA or any other hormone? A good way to find out is through testing. Saliva tests and blood tests are available to determine your level of DHEA, growth hormone, and melatonin, as well as other hormones.

You can contact clinical laboratories, mentioned in our web site, or other clinical reference labs that offer this testing as well.

A good rule of thumb is to compare your blood DHEA level to that of a thirty-year-old, which is about 200 mcg/d to 300 mcg/d in the blood for females and 300 mcg/d to 400 mcg/d in the males. Saliva tests have their own reference ranges. You may want to retest yourself every three months, then every six months to make sure you are still in the reference range of a person thirty years of age. Consult an integrative medicine endocrinologist for recommendations.

I covered these last three hormones individually because I think they are probably the most important hormones in an anti-aging hormone replacement program. Melatonin establishes set points for your biological clock and may influence the declining levels of all your other hormones as you age.

Sex and Hormones

Do you recall when you first learned how babies were made? Depending on your age, the news was either confusing or "Yuck! How gross." Later on you realized that when your parents locked the bedroom door, "They-Were-Doing-It." The whole idea was so . . . so . . . Yech! It made you want to gag. You looked at them the next morning, wondering if Doing It showed on their faces. Suddenly they embarrassed you.

As you got closer to your teens you began looking at the opposite sex with more than some curiosity. And then with some desire. And you didn't give much thought to what Mom and Dad were doing behind that closed door. Once you were an adult and sexually active there was no stopping you or your constant thoughts, especially if you were a man.

Later still, you may have settled down to a life with a spouse and children, and eventually sex became a perfunctory event. Lust was still present occasionally, but for the most part, you were too busy to do anything about it anyway.

Now, you're older. The kids are gone. Maybe your spouse has deceased. For some of you, your libido got up and went, too. Sex is the farthest thing from your mind. All this talk about Viagra . . . well, it doesn't mean anything to you. You're just as happy not having to do it at all. In fact, the idea of getting naked and having sex at your age makes you snicker. Makes you want to gag.

Note that I said "for some of you," since there are others among you for whom sex is still a great and pleasurable pastime.

People who continue sexual activity into older age, assuming a hale and hearty lifestyle in other respects, will, according to research, probably live the longest.

Sexuality is healthy and helps us enjoy our life experience through all our later ages. If you feel attractive, you feel better about yourself. Sexual activity, reduces stress and probably increases life. There's a reason for that. Sex with a loving partner is a great hormone stimulant. If you suppress a natural hormone enhancer, after a while the hormone stops being produced. It goes back to the Use It or Lose It Principle.

Who has the greater sexual energy? Teenagers and people in their twenties, up to their early thirties. Who has sex most often? Teenagers, people in their twenties, and up to their early thirties.

So at what level do we want to maintain our hormones? To the level of a thirty or maybe a forty-year-old?

And what stimulates a cascade of hormone production from cholesterol to pregnenolone to DHEA, on and on, to estrogen and testosterone?

Sexual activity is a natural stimulant for hormone production, just like physical activity.

Recently I saw an 82-year-old female patient that truly impressed me with her charm, keen interest in life, wit, energy and sultry sexuality. She looked 25 years younger, the skin on her belly was smooth and soft like a 40 year old, and her face looked like a young sixty year old. She dressed attractively, and in a subtle way, flirted with me and her much younger companion who had a keen interest in her. To me this 82 year old lady was sexy. She was more charming and flirtatious than most 45-year old patients that I have seen. I wondered why this lady was so different from the others? After completing my extensive history the reasons for her youth were clear, she had been taking female hormone replacements for two months before her hysterectomy at age 42 as well as taking lots of natural vitamins along with being physically active.

The hormones, vitamins, and physical activity kept her young physically, sexually and mentally.

Sex at an older age is an important spark in lighting the fire that keeps you young and healthy. Sex stimulates all the other hormones and gets the adrenaline pumping, as well as giving you considerable pleasure and intimacy. You'll benefit by staying sharper and having clearer thinking without that short-term memory loss that most aging people suffer. Sex rounds out your life and gives you an overall glow and radiance that I don't see in old fuddy-duddies. The cuddling alone is so valuable for your wellbeing.

You've heard the term, grumpy old men. Maybe with increased sexual activity, we'd have fewer grumpy and *younger* old men. This may sound preposterous, but it makes biological sense. Let's go over the biological hormonal rationale of what I am saying.

Just as music and art stimulate the brain and keep the connectors working and sprouting new ones, so too does sexual activity, producing emotional and hormonal well-being.

In the calorically-restricted mice studies, the mice that were calorically restricted were sexually active well into old age, and although chronologically old when they died, were biologically young.

On observations of people who were calorically restricted, I have noticed, from their comments, that not only were they a little bit hungry all the time, they were also a little bit horny. To me, that means the hormones are working at a younger level than your age, helping to keep you youthful.

Older men who had decreased sex drives, softened muscles, and increased fat used testosterone to increase their libidos. In a study at

Emory University, thirteen elderly men were given testosterone for three months and compared to men receiving placebos. The men who received testosterone developed increased muscle mass, less bone mineral loss, reduced overall cholesterol levels, and best of all, increased sex drives. Those men who took the testosterone patches noticed an increased sexual excitability, as well as competency. Another beneficial side effect had been that they were less depressed.

The problem with using testosterone externally is that it may result in undesirable effects, such as possibly stimulating prostatic tumors or increasing the production of red blood cells and therefore thickening the blood and making you a greater risk for stroke. This is where all the blood thinning vitamins and leafy green vegetables come in handy. Some people also take a baby aspirin to thin their blood.

Natural stimulation of testosterone through sexual arousal is preferable to synthetic application of the patch.

Simultaneously, it's not just the men who benefit from increased sexual activity. Women do, too.

Did you know that while the stress hormone cortisol can be destructive to neurons, estrogen is protective of neurons? It was noted, earlier, that women who have had their ovaries removed (and therefore lacked estrogen) began complaining of memory loss.

Researchers started looking at memory and estrogen and found that estrogen is important in preserving women's memories by helping to regulate neuronal communications through the increased density of those branching root-like fibers in the brain, known as dendrites. Sexual activity stimulates estrogen just as it does the other sex hormones.

Barbara Sherwin, a Canadian researcher, noticed these findings and began giving memory tests to women before their gynecological surgery, while they still had adequate estrogen levels. She then re-tested them again after their ovaries were removed.

She found that after the surgery, the women's mental skills declined. However, those who were given estrogen replacement regained their mental skills to the pre-surgical state. The mental skills of those who did not receive the estrogen remained at a declined level. What you see is a common problem of aging, decreased mental acuity.

Did you know that Alzheimer's disease is twice as common in women as men? Have you ever considered that the postmenopausal drop in the estrogen level may be partly to blame for that memory loss? If you are highly stressed and producing high levels of cortisol and not producing estrogen, you're getting a double whammy.

You are destroying your brain cells, and at the same time not nourishing them and preserving them. I don't want to linger on such a devastating disease as Alzheimer's, which takes more than a 100,000 lives a year, but we must understand that estrogens are not only important for sexual behavior and activity, but they are also important in learning, memory and neuronal preservation.

A recent study at the National Institute on Aging, women were given estrogen replacement and found there was a 50% reduction in the development of Alzheimer's disease. Other researchers found that estrogen exhibits antioxidant, as well as anti-inflammatory, activities and helps neuronal growth, which in turn increases the neurotransmitters that are so important for brain communication.

I have talked about the Use It or Lose It Principle with brain stimulation. Here we have another example where the lack of an important hormone is implicated in memory loss. This boosts my theory even more that constant stimulation of estrogen, for those women who did not have a total abdominal hysterectomy, will increase their hormone level and therefore maintain and preserve their cognitive function. If you had a total abdominal hysterectomy try to get natural hormonal replacement.

The more I think about it, sexual activity and sexual desire may be an important anti-aging biomarker. It is dependent upon adequate and healthy blood flow, as well as adequate hormones in your circulation to start the arousal cascade.

Just as your sex life may be an indicator of the overall compatibility and health of your marriage, your sexual interests and performance may also be an indicator of your overall aging status.

Through my personal observation, I have seen that older individuals with increased sexual interest and performance are younger in appearance, stamina, and more interested in the world around them.

If you follow the basic premise of this book, "Use It or Lose It," sexual activity is another component in maintaining your youth. If you can practice doing the things you did when you were younger, you'll get better at them.

Sexual activity will make you feel younger, give you more energy, enhance your muscular strength, improve your circulation and help maintain your brain neurons by constant estrogen and testosterone stimulation.

Just Do It! You'll be glad you did.

Other Hormones

Throughout my medical career, I have been a proponent of the natural approach on the road to maintaining health. Whenever there was a non-drug alternative that had potentially the same benefits as that of a proprietary drug, I told my patients to use that alternative first, unless a drug was absolutely necessary in order, for example, to treat a massive infection. I'm sure you've heard of people dying of pneumonia because they refused to get medical care. Traditional medicine, sometimes, is the only way to go. It certainly comes in handy in an emergency.

Due to the booming pharmaceutical industry (approximately 130 billion dollars a year globally), a lot of natural approaches toward healing have been suppressed. Natural agents that have similar effects to drugs are, generally, not known among physicians because they aren't informed about them.

Natural agents don't provide free dinners or monetary remunerations for experimental trial studies. Natural agents don't make money for hospitals.

They also don't cost $75.00 a pill.

In many parts of the world, nontoxic, natural therapeutics are the treatments of choice before more invasive pharmacological intervention is taken.

A German systematic study of herbs was published in a report entitled "The Complete German Commission Monographs Therapeutic Guide to Herbal Medicines". The report was reprinted in English by the American Botanical Counsel. The many therapeutic benefits of herbs were outlined and extensively studied. How many American doctors do you think knew anything about this?

The problem, I realize, is that American medicine and the pharmaceutical industry are overly busy trying to make money and corporate profits rather than trying to improve health. The only anti-aging products you will ever hear about from the pharmaceutical industry are the ones they can synthetically produce and patent and that show great potential for profit. Recently, however, pharmaceutical companies have started buying up vitamin companies because so many people use vitamins now.

It is your responsibility to educate yourself on how you can prolong your healthy life and live longer.

This reminds me of my favorite aunt in Germany, who is in her eighties, and a pharmacist. Her husband and daughter are also pharmacists. My aunt was always a botanist and proponent of natural teas and herbs for the treatment of various diseases. She used to know just about every plant that grew in the meadows and forests, and their health-healing properties.

I saw Aunt Eva recently and she is still as sharp as a tack. She had a great influence on me in looking at nature for cures in human ailments. Her garden was always full of many varieties of plants that I never heard of, and she would use them for medicinal purposes.

There are well over 100 hormones in your body. While I can't discuss every hormone and its purpose, there are a few that are worth mentioning since they do affect your overall well-being. Did you know that your thyroid hormone is very important to how you feel? An underactive thyroid can cause a large number of symptoms which initially seem unrelated. The thyroid hormone also decreases with age, and periodic monitoring of it should be performed by your doctor to have optimal health.

The thyroid gland is right in the front of your throat by your Adam's apple. It is involved in energy production, growth, temperature regulation, colds, allergies, blood circulation, metabolism, fat deposit, immunity, waste product removal, wound healing, hair loss, headaches, irregular heart rhythms, and a host of other conditions you may never have associated with it, including memory problems and hardening of the arteries.

Generally, women are more afflicted with hypothyroidism, about seven to eight times more. The older you are, the greater your chance of hypothyroidism. If you are diabetic, you may also be susceptible to this disease. If you are taking certain medications, such as beta-blockers or lithium, that may also affect your thyroid.

If you are also deficient in certain trace elements, such as iodine, iron, zinc, or selenium, you may have impairment in converting one type of thyroid hormone, called T3, into the T4 active form. Also, if you are deficient in vitamins A, E, or riboflavin, or certain amino acids such as cysteine, you may develop hypothyroidism. If you lack fats in your diet or are malnourished, have growth hormone deficiencies, or lack melatonin or insulin, hypothyroidism may develop.

Hypothyroidism can also be caused by substances we rarely think about, such as excessive intake of iodine through some drugs, or kelp, or even antibiotics, or prolonged use of tetracycline for acne treatment, or nitrates. If you have had radiation treatment to the neck and face, you may also suffer from hypothyroidism.

Generally, if you are a woman older than forty, or a man older than sixty-five, you are more prone to hypothyroidism. If you feel cold all the time, fatigued, have anxiety or panic attacks, or are chronically depressed, have headaches, hair loss, dry skin, brittle hair, thinning hair, brittle or weak nails, shortness of breath, menstruation problems, infertility, miscarriages, or swelling, have yourself checked for thyroid deficiency.

Some people may also develop hyperthyroidism through lithium, high fat diets, high protein diets, or hormonal excesses such as cortisol--the stress hormone, as well as certain medications and toxins, such as excessive use of alcohol. This is a tricky hormone that can mimic other diseases. It should be monitored as part of your regular blood work.

Pregnenolone is a precursor to DHEA, as I mentioned previously. The good thing about it is that it is a great hormone to be taken in stressful situations and in situations where you have to be mentally sharp. Pregnenolone is a neuro-enhancer, as well as a mood enhancer, and it just makes you feel good. The best thing about it is that it is extremely safe compared to other things you may take. If you want to take it in conjunction with DHEA, for its anti-aging effect, besides its mood enhancement and antiinflammatory and anti-arthritic effect, it may not be a bad idea.

Many women request hormone replacement therapy after they reach menopause. You may consider consulting physicians trained in natural hormone replacement. The benefits of natural hormones are that they have both fewer side effects and more positive biological action.

The reasons you may want to have natural hormone replacement are to maintain a high quality of life, prevent osteoporosis, heart disease, Alzheimer's disease, and as previously discussed, with the increased estrogen level, relief from the effects of menopause. You also want to avoid the increased risk of acquiring the various cancers that have been associated with various synthetic hormones.

Doctors who are practitioners in natural hormone replacement recommend estriol (E3), which is milder and much gentler than its synthetic equivalent because it fails to occupy the estrogen receptors for a prolonged period, thus reducing side effects.

Natural micronized progesterone is preferable to the synthetic progestin (which is found in birth control pills and is frequently prescribed by physicians). Synthetic progestin may lead to thrombophlebitis, pulmonary emboli, fluid retention, seizures, weight gain, elevated blood pressure, depression, hair loss, and so forth. Therefore, natural micronized progesterone is the treatment of choice for many physicians practicing in natural hormone replacement. The usual dosage is 100 to 200 mg per day. Progesterone cream has been used successfully to relieve hot flashes.

Natural testosterone is also used to help improve sex lives, as well as a sense of wellbeing and vigor, and may also improve muscle strength, help increase bone density, and help reduce urinary incontinence. It is given in doses of 1 mg to 10 mg a day.

As I mentioned, previously, when individual hormone replacement therapy is undertaken, it needs to be done very slowly and gradually, and it needs to be monitored by a capable physician. I recommend looking at the Website of the American College for the Advancement of Medicine at *www.acam.org* and search the qualifications of the physicians in your area to see if they practice natural hormone replacement therapy.

NADH

Many of you may never have heard of this co-enzyme. Others may even wonder why I am including this in the hormone section. I'm doing this because it has a mixed variety of benefits, which I think should be included in a longevity program.

NADH, which is called nicotinamide adenine dinucleotide, is very important for energy production in every cell of our bodies. Because of that, it is also a potent anti-aging substance. NADH is actually the fuel for our cells which produce energy known as ATP. As a matter of fact, one molecule of NADH produces three molecules of ATP.

All of this may sound foreign to you, but ATP is nothing but the pure energy that our cells use to survive and do things. NADH also plays a role in cell regulation and repair of our DNA molecules, which is the make-up of everything in our body. It enhances our immune system, and is an extremely potent antioxidant. Another interesting fact about NADH is that it stimulates neurotransmitters such as dopamine, norepinephrine, adrenaline, and enhances their production.

What does all this mean? It means you have a substance that is capable of repairing damaged DNA in our cells, a substance that enhances our immune system, and a substance that is an extremely potent antioxidant. As a matter of fact, it is a stronger antioxidant than glutathione, which I had mentioned previously. Both NADH and glutathione are being used to treat Parkinson's Disease. There have been several clinical trials completed in Europe and in the United States with beneficial results. By its stimulation of adrenaline and dopamine (which are lacking in Parkinson's patients), it helps coordinate strength and movement, alertness, cognition, and mood, as well as stimulate growth hormone and a sex drive.

John P. Lenhart M.D.

Dopamine is known to be important in all sectors of the sex drive including ejaculation, orgasm, and so forth.

Another beneficial effect of NADH is that by increasing dopamine and adrenaline in your system, you have less of an appetite and can control your weight more efficiently. It has also been reported that NADH protects the liver from alcohol damage. It enables testosterone production, which is important, even if you have alcohol in your system. Usually alcohol inhibits testosterone production.

NADH lowers cholesterol levels as well as blood pressure, helps with depression, and studies have found it to be helpful in Alzheimer's disease and other dementias in which there is a loss of memory and deterioration of the activities of daily living. NADH has also shown promising benefits in combatting chronic fatigue syndrome by supplying energy to the cells. It's a fairly interesting co-enzyme.

The thing I like most about it is that it is extremely safe. Even at very high concentrations, side effects have not been noticed. The dosage of NADH that has been used is 5 mg a day. However, even much higher doses than that have been well tolerated.

One word of caution: NADH breaks down very rapidly in pill form, so get it in a micronized form. It is essential that it remains stable after a prolonged shelf life so that you can benefit from it. You need to be very careful of the kind you get. It is also available in IV solutions.

Since it is such a powerful anti-oxidant and is essential in energy production, NADH should be considered in your longevity armament.

As you can see from this chapter, hormones can be very complicated. Personally, I don't think the medical world understands the full interactive and interdependent applications of hormones.

We are currently at a stage in medicine where we are trying to kill a fly on the wall with a shotgun and there are a lot of other victims besides the fly. There is a lot that we do not know about our bodies' molecular intricacies. It is, therefore, pertinent that you remain cautious when testing out new hormone replacements, and make sure that the hormones are taken in their most natural form. If possible, use a hormone replacement with the exact molecular formula of the original.

For example, in human growth hormone, the first version lacked one of the amino acids. However, in 1986, Ely Lily produced Humatrope, which was exactly the same as natural growth hormone.

The body is not very tolerant of imitators, even if they are close. Some of the hormones I mentioned are fairly safe and are precursors to a myriad other hormones. They are like the snow that produces those snowballs, where the body itself decides at which balanced ratios the other hormones will be produced.

With natural hormones, you will have specific hormones produced at safer levels and that are more easily tolerated by your system. These hormones are gentle and reduce the issue of over-stimulating the other hormones in your body.

This is a broad topic, and those of you who are further interested in hormone replacement should read books dedicated to that field. Hormones play an important part in anti-aging, from setting your biological clock to promoting growth and tranquility and stabilizing your brain/nerve cells. Hormones are also important in energy production and affect your overall sense of well-being.

The more naturally you can increase hormones, the better, such as through vigorous physical exercise, as previously discussed. However, sometimes supplementation is needed. If you decide to use high dosages of hormone precursors, I recommend having your hormone levels monitored, either by blood tests or saliva tests, and also have your intake monitored by a qualified physician.

Now for the bad news: Researchers have very recently discovered a "switch" in the round worm, a commonly studied species. Once the reproductive phase is over, this switch turns on which starts the aging process. In humans it's the decrease of growth hormone, estrogen, testosterone and other hormones. The Telomeres on our chromosomes get shorter, we get shorter, our mind gets filled up with tangles and so on. Every cell in our body has programmed cell death, called apoptosis. For every action there is an equal and opposite reaction, a law of Physics. Be careful what you put into your body and mind.

My goal in this book is to get you stimulated to start your healthy aging and longevity journey. You never get anywhere unless you take the first step and start. I want every fellow baby boomer to have the best retirement possible and to enjoy the fruits of their labor without physical impediments.

CHAPTER 8

Fruits, Vegetables, and Dietary Choices

Hippocrates said "Let food be thy medicine and let medicine be thy food," You have to ask yourself is the food we eat today really food?

You are what you eat, and in this chapter I hope to at least nudge you towards making wiser choices in what you put into your body. It is good to know why you are doing something, instead of just taking some magic pill that you know nothing about. Every human body is slightly different. This is the only body that we have, so we had better make sure we give it the best building blocks possible in order for it to grow healthy and repair itself when things go wrong.

After listening to the Shenandoah Park Rangers give their talks, I noticed that the topics they covered about Nature had direct implications for this book.

Shenandoah National Park in Virginia used to have Peregrine Falcons. Over the past dozen years they slowly disappeared from the park and no one knew why.

After prolonged study, it was determined that the DDT-sprayed crops eaten by insects and then eaten by small birds, who in turn were eaten by the falcons, was the culprit. The DDT-infested prey of the Falcons caused their egg shells to be thin and break easily. Without strong egg shells the young hatching chicks could not survive as they broke while being laid or due to the elements. No new Falcons were being born, and the species became extinct in the park.

After DDT was banned, new falcons were introduced into the park. According to the park rangers, only one pair, so far, has stayed and reproduced with its offspring remaining in the park. It is much harder to get something back after you lose it. The same is true with our health, as pointed out in chapter 4, in the Physical Activity and Exercise chapter.

This is a perfect example of the harmful repercussions of chemicals in our food that we may not even be aware of. Throughout my recent travels I would see many pesticide-spray tractors, with large booms on either side spraying the crops, as well as crop duster airplanes buzzing overhead. I couldn't help wondering how this spraying might be affecting our future generations. Did you ever wonder why "Low T" has become such a big business? Are men really producing less testosterone nowadays? How is this going to affect our great, great, grandkids? The food we eat today does have an effect on future generations. Remember that epigenetics research that was done in Scandinavia where they kept accurate records of past generations?

This chapter on Dietary choices is important because it gives you guidelines on how to select healthy foods that may affect your health in the future.

As I watched a program on PBS about the damming of the Little Colorado River to make Lake Powell I noticed similarities in the ecological changes that have occurred in that river and its habitats to what happens in the human body.

You see, the scientists for the Department of Natural Resources had only looked at the Little Colorado; its course through the Grand Canyon was their lone concern. What would happen to the river upstream where the area was dammed up?

They gave no thought, also, to the changes five miles, ten miles, or even fifty miles downstream. They didn't realize that the creation of a dam and alteration of the water flow would change the natural fish populations and their distributions. The scientists only started questioning that when they noticed the native fish populations dying off and invasive fish increasing in numbers. On that PBS program, they admitted they had looked at the river as small segments instead of the one big entity it was; they failed to take note that a change upstream would affect the habitats of species a hundred miles downstream.

So they decided to push the system out of equilibrium a little bit further, and create a small flood, called the Grand Canyon flood, to see if they could change the environment back to its original natural habitat. Well, guess what happened?

Large boulders eroded off the banks, entire beaches disappeared, new sediments appeared at other parts of the river, and the fish and wildlife species had to, more or less, adapt to this temporary change in the water flow.

The scientists knew there would be erosion. After all, look at the Grand Canyon, a master example of the power of water reshaping landscape with its deep canyons and rainbow-colored vistas. At the end of their mini-flood experiment, the scientists marveled and said, "Nature is not easily led or dominated." It has resilience, but entire species of animals and plants can be totally wiped out just by changing the balanced equilibrium.

Just think about our colon, when we wipe out entire species of native organisms through excessive antibiotic use, the landscape is no longer the same. New organisms pop up that are not natural to our gut environment, and beneficial intestinal bacteria are annihilated.

Water changed the Colorado River landscape forever, just as it changed our ecological equilibriums.

In the human body, we call this equilibrium homeostasis, meaning maintaining things in balance. As the Little Colorado River's landscape, wildlife, and banks are influenced by the boulders rolling down with the river's force, along with the grasses, vegetation and banks being altered, so, too, our body reacts in a similar way by what goes through it.

The type of water we drink has a vast effect on every single chemical reaction that exists in our body. The more polluted and unnatural the water is, the greater will be the stress that eventually erodes our body and causes deep furrows like the Grand Canyon. Over time this causes permanent scars affecting our biological equilibrium. Like the altered shoreline and erosion formed from the flooding in the Grand Canyon, our body's biological pattern will also change if we allow foreign substances, such as unnatural, chemically polluted water into it.

The debris we accumulate through our water, and foods, makes it nearly impossible for our biological interactions to work properly, or the blood to flow smoothly throughout our vessels without eddies and rapids of their own, eventually leading to arteriosclerosis and our demise through stroke, heart attack, or senility.

Yes, ladies and gentlemen, it all starts with the water.

Our bodies are made up of between fifty and seventy percent water. If you have a lot of fat, it is closer to fifty percent; if you're lean, it's closer to seventy percent. Water is an essential component in every cell in our bodies.

Water is required for nutrient transfer to our cells. It is important for our brain cells to work, our lungs to work, and our entire absorption system of foods. Our muscles, including our heart, would stop working without adequate water. Because we lose water through respiration (breathing) and perspiration, as well as urination, we would survive only a few days without a constant supply.

One good thing is that the body constantly changes itself and you have a chance of rebuilding yourself every year. Did you know that your red blood cells only last about four months? That's right, you have all new blood every one hundred and twenty days. You lose 50 million skin cells per day and develop a new gut lining every 10 days. I have read that your entire body recycles itself about every seven years. All these chemical reactions are dependent on water since water is the perfect solvent that allows us to transfer minerals and nutrients, as well as vitamins, into our cells. But all is not well in the water world.

Contamination with toxic chemicals, fertilizers, and additives has made our water dangerously polluted, to the point where it can interfere with our body's enzymatic pathways, as well as its normal metabolism. These interferences can cause massive stress on our body, which eventually wears down our repair mechanisms and we get catastrophic diseases, such as cancer, senility, cardiovascular disease, and so on.

Take plastic water bottles, for instance. What may be a seemingly harmless way to distribute water to millions may be doing more harm than good to our bodies. I once read a report which stated that one part per million of a toxic chemical, of which we have many in our normal drinking water, produces six-hundred-quadrillion toxic molecules. That is 600, plus 15 zeros. That's a heck of a lot of toxic molecules that could be interfering with our normal cell function, and could eventually lead to cell death, abnormal replication, or just tired, worn-out cells that are tired of fighting these chemicals.

One significant thing, substances such as chlorine and fluoride are sometimes added to water, which are known to cause major health problems. Chlorine is added to kill off dangerous bacteria. However, when chlorine is combined with organic substances, you end up with chlorinated hydrocarbons, a toxin to the body, which may cause hardening of the arteries, heart attacks, and other age-related diseases.

As I recounted earlier, when I went to Memorial University in Newfoundland to talk to the lead researcher in the Canadian Longevity Aging Study, I found that no one was there and that they had shut that part of the university down for a day because of unacceptable high levels of lead in the drinking water in several buildings. They were trying to find the source of this toxic heavy metal. Do you know what's in your water?

There is a book written by Dr. John Yiamouyiannis, titled *Fluoride, The Aging Factor*. He documents how fluoride alters the body's production of collagen, which is the connective tissue between the cells and our joints, as well as affecting our arteries and our skin. Remember all that plaque buildup inside our arteries? Well, it can only build up if the arteries are not smooth and are partially damaged.

He also points out that fluoride can cause autoimmune disease and alterations in our DNA repair mechanisms, which make up the building blocks of our genes and cells. Did you ever wonder how DNA starts mutating, leading to uncontrolled growth? There has to be a trigger or multiple triggers.

Just think about it. Forty years ago, would you have thought that people would make a profit selling water? European bottled water was sold to high end, fancy-shmansy people that only bought it for the high mineral content. Later on, you started seeing water machines in supermarkets. Now, there is bottled water everywhere, mostly sold in plastic.

Why are people buying bottled water when they can be drinking it free out of the tap? Because the majority of the people are much smarter than you think. They realize that you have to start with something pure, especially if it is a solvent in all the other foods you eat, allows you to absorb everything, and helps to filter out all the waste through your kidneys.

The contaminants that are around us don't stop with water, either. We thought we would do a good job in cleaning up our air by putting catalytic converters on our cars and changing the gasoline to make it lead-free. Well, they put an additive into our gasoline called MTBE, which is so darn toxic that it infiltrates the ground water and has been found in varying amounts in all fifty states.

A European study linked MTBE to liver and kidney tumors in mice. While we have clean-burning gasoline with this stuff, we're being poisoned internally. You figure it out. Maybe that's why everyone is buying bottled water.

I'll go one step further, distilled water. Distilled water combined with a charcoal filter removes just about all the impurities. You are left with a perfect solvent for dissolving your organic minerals and nutrients, bathing yourself internally with clean, pure water that will not change its chemical consistency or produce mutations due to its toxic load. Many of my arthritis patients drink distilled water to help alleviate the arthritic symptoms. You see, it all starts with water.

Most of us assume that the food and water we drink is safe for consumption. After all we have the FDA in the USA to look out for us, right? Think again. In 2015 a series of articles came out about Marines that lived at the marine base in Camp Lejeune North Carolina. Researchers noticed that they had a higher than normal rate of male breast cancer. Breast cancer is not usually associated with men. As researchers looked into the issue, there was a startling realization that the water supply may have been contaminated with small doses of discarded petroleum products. So, how safe is our water?

During my travels, I ran into a fellow RVer traveling solo in a small Class B motorhome like mine. When I interviewed this lady, I found out that she was an independent thinker from northern California, willing to stick her neck out and explore the world. When our conversation got to doctors, I learned that she rarely goes to them. The last time she went she was told that she had hypothyroidism and would need to take thyroid hormone. She researched it and, instead, decided to start drinking distilled water and eating more fruits and vegetables and no processed food. Guess what? She told me that when she returned to the doctor to get re-tested, her thyroid had returned to normal.

Some of you may be saying, "I heard that distilled water is bad for you because it doesn't have any minerals." Let me answer that.

The minerals that you absorb from food are organic minerals. That means they have been absorbed in their organic shape from the ground, through vegetables and fruits, and transformed into a food that we can use biologically. We don't have the same mechanisms as plants to transform inorganic minerals to organic minerals. We may have a little bit of an ability to do that, but it's minimal compared to the benefits we get from eating organic minerals through vegetables and fruits. Maybe that's why some of those vitamin/mineral studies came back negative because they contained non-bioavailable inorganic minerals.

If you can't afford a distiller for your house, then maybe a reverse osmosis system would be the next best thing. It has a very high filtration rate through the micropore membranes through which the water is squeezed. There are other forms of cartridge filters around, which are good; however, the distillation process and the reverse osmosis system are probably the best.

Did you know that distilled water even enhances your mineral absorption rate? The reason distilled water is used in car batteries is to keep the lead plates from breaking down as fast. Distilled water will not conduct electricity when two parts inorganic minerals or less are present.

Just think about it, distilled water has two parts inorganic minerals or less, while the average American tap water ranges between 350 to 1000 parts per million of contaminants. Remember that one part per million created six-hundred-quadrillion toxic molecules. I think you are starting to get the picture.

The purer the water, the less contamination you get into your body.

I have always found it interesting how the safety of toxins such as aluminum, arsenic, chloride, cobalt, lead, or even nitrates is measured. . Researchers generally feed this stuff to animals and find out at what level 50% of them die. Pretty scientific, huh?

Well, they can't feed it to humans so they have to give it to rats, or mice or guinea pigs, or something like that. Then, they come out with a statement ". . . This chemical is safe at so many parts per million." Okay, I'll buy that.

Then they do another study with another chemical that they decide to use, such as, let's say, aspartame, or anything like that, and they say, "Okay we can take so much of that and it doesn't cause any problems right now. Of course, we don't know if it will cause any problems five generations down the line, but right now, it doesn't cause any problems." Have they heard of the science of epigenetics (how our inherited genes can be altered by external switches)? What we do in our reproductive years influences the health of several generations down the line.

They take another chemical, do the same thing, and eventually if you read the label on a jar of stuff you buy, it has thirty different chemicals in it. You buy another product, and it has twenty different chemicals. You eat in a restaurant where they use normal tap water run through lead pipes and that has a whole slew of its own chemicals. Then you go outside and breathe the exhaust of the cars whizzing by. In large cities you have another whole set of polluting chemicals, which your lungs absorb, you know that stuff they call smog.

Then you go into your office building and it has what is known as Sick Building Syndrome. On your way home from the office, the lawn has just been sprayed with some kind of organophosphate fertilizer or maybe even a pesticide, and you get a whiff of that. By the time you get home, you may have accumulated a hefty dose of chemicals which have been deemed "safe" individually, but in combination and cumulatively, they may play major havoc on your immune system and your ability to age in a healthy manner.

You see, the constant flow of chemicals that we expose ourselves to day after day are slowly breaking us down, putting toxins in our body that we cannot detoxify effectively as those toxins did not exist when we were first evolving. This toxic stress reaches a point where the cells just cannot handle it anymore, and you start getting sick, very, very sick.

Is that the way you want to live? In this toxic environment? The title of this book is *Happy Life Healthy Aging*. Living with toxic water does not lead to healthy aging. Get out of that pollution, and start drinking pure healthy water.

I was reading a recent article from the Associated Press, entitled "Lymphoma Rise Baffling, But New Therapies in Sight." It stated that this mysterious immune system cancer has been making a quiet comeback and rates have nearly doubled since the seventies. It questioned if diet was to blame, or whether pesticides, air pollution, viruses, or obesity were factors. As the article says, nobody knows, and they will be launching major studies to discover what's behind the rapid rise of this type of cancer.

Well, it is a cancer of the immune system and obviously we are taking something internally that is decreasing our resistance. We might say that we are not taking enough of the right nutrients internally to increase our resistance. Just as I stated before, "Garbage in, garbage out."

People are fortifying their immune systems as if they are building paper houses. Any wind that comes along will blow that house over. More and more people are becoming aware of the potential dangers of pesticides, chemicals, heavy metal toxicity, GMOs (genetically modified organisms), and are demanding organically grown foods. Vermont was the first state to require labeling of bioengineered ingredients. However, restaurants, which provide one third of all calories consumed, were exempted.

The U.S. Federal Government is attempting to define and regulate organic foods, by defining "organic" as something that does not have genetically modified ingredients, is not irradiated to decontaminate the product, and sewage sludge has not been utilized as fertilizer. This is just a minor start in an avalanche of future discovery that the food we consume is slowly poisoning us. Why did it take so long for artery-clogging trans fats to be banned from our food chain? If you see a label saying partially hydrogenated fats, they are trans fats.

Walter Willett, chairman of the department of nutrition at Harvard University's school of public health stated, "This was really the biggest food processing disaster ever. The human toll has got to be in the millions."

Partially hydrogenated oils have been used since the 1940's because they made food last longer. Initially, they were thought to be safer than natural saturated fats such as butter. Ever wonder why pastries would last forever? Why do processed foods such as packaged cookies, crackers, cakes, soft buns, pizza dough, vegetable shortening, hard margarine, pre mixes such as frostings, pancake mix, chocolate mix, French fries, tortilla, corn and potato chips, chicken nuggets, snack foods, microwave popcorn and soft breads last a long time? It's due to the trans fats found in them.

The food industry loved trans fats. They increased the shelf life of food and made the food cheaper to produce. Fast food chains only recently banned trans fats from their products. How long have we been eating these artery clogging products? Remember that friendly neighbor, the food industry, that leaves things at your home (your body), and slowly clogs up your house with chemical toxins?

It took a lawsuit in 2015 from a 100 year old scientist, Dr. Fred Kummerow, a University of Illinois professor, to finally get the FDA to put a ban on these products. He had been researching trans fats for 60 years and warning about their dangers in clogging up the arteries. He was able to develop arterioclerosis in rats by giving them trans fats. When the trans fats were removed from the rats' diet, the arteriosclerosis went away.

This is an excellent example of how the friendly foods that we have been eating may slowly be killing us. I noticed this at the northern Newfoundland Labrador area with the epidemic level of childhood obesity there.

Talking to knowledgeable people in the area, community nurses, doctors, and social workers, the problem occurred when children started eating fast foods. Computers, computer games, lack of exercise and the sedentary lifestyle have also contributed to this childhood obesity epidemic. It was rare for me to see a thin teenager in that region. You would think an area that specializes in fishing would have healthy people, but that was not what I found. The social worker at a long-term-care home told me that she is seeing younger and younger people coming into her facility.

Where was our government in all these years while we've been slowly getting poisoned by this processed artificially enhanced food we've been eating?

The major food companies aren't standing still now. They see money to be made in natural foods and they're all jumping into the arena. For example, Nestle USA joined the natural and functional food niche with the introduction of dietary supplements. H. J. Heinz Company also formed an organic and nutritional food unit. Quaker Oats, another large company, got involved in the functional food business, which is designed to offer specific health benefits above basic nutrition.

Did you know that General Mills, Inc., Kraft Foods, Inc., and Kellogg's Company have all gotten into this wellness arena, and that they have been gobbling up smaller companies that have been in the health food industry for some time?

We have companies specializing in unprocessed organic foods springing up all over the place. Even the major grocery chains have organic sections now.

What's happening is as the consumers, especially the baby-boomers, become savvy about pesticides and genetically modified foods, they search out the health benefits of foods in order to live longer.

The baby-boomers want to stay healthy and active into old age and they know that food has something to do with the disease processes we are all experiencing. The big companies, sensing a market, are all getting into it.

Sales within the organic and natural food industry have grown fifteen to twenty percent per year, compared to one to two percent for general grocery merchandising. In Europe, where they have massive protests against genetically engineered foods, sales of natural foods are growing even faster. Europeans have always been health-oriented and they're rebelling against artificial ingredients, preferring pure, unadulterated sources as building blocks for cells.

All this change in the food industry is good for you, the consumer. It is going to create greater competition and a larger selection of healthy foods that you can buy. Since the government is going to be regulating it to a certain extent, we hope that they will have more and more rules in the future, but it is a good start in the right direction.

Maybe, someday, you will be able to get a choice of supplements as your after-dinner treat at a fancy restaurant instead of the traditional mint to help you digest your food. They may still be mint-flavored, however they'll be designed to nutritionally augment and balance the food you just consumed. Is this Utopia or is this a possibility?

Talking about utopia, I'm rewriting this chapter on spectacular Marble Mountain, in southern Cape Breton Island, Nova Scotia, Canada. There is an overlook rest stop high above the absolutely gorgeous Bras d' Or Lake, a UNESCO biosphere Reserve. When I say spectacular, I mean spectacular with fluffy clouds, distant islands and breathtaking views. The closest places in the USA with similar views that I have been to are Crater Lake Oregon and the Waterton-Glacier International Peace Park World Heritage Site at the Montana USA Alberta Canada border.

Recently, I was traveling in Sopot, Poland. While at a walk-in clinic, I noticed that the doctor on call would prescribe antibiotics and then follow with a prescription of vitamins and probiotic bacteria to replenish the ones destroyed by the antibiotics. Now that's progressive integrative medicine.

Let's get down to earth and discuss what you can do to get the best nutrients possible in the foods you eat. While you have always heard the saying that you should be eating at least five servings of fruits and vegetables per day, to be divided by three servings of vegetables and two of fruit, how do you choose?

I like to think of it as a beautiful rainbow going over the water, and there is a pot of gold at the end of that rainbow. But, the trick is, you have to eat the rainbow to reach the pot of gold. Just as bees and various insects are attracted to colors in fruit for pollination, we should be attracted to colors in vegetables and fruits for sustentation. Generally, the brighter the color of something, the more vitamins and minerals it has to enhance our health. The duller the food, the less nutrients it has.

So what are the colors of the rainbow? Red, orange, yellow, green, blue, indigo, violet... beautiful colors. What foods can you think of that follow that rainbow scheme?

Let's start with red. Think hard, what is red. I know it's on the tip of your tongue. How about tomatoes, cherries, strawberries, cranberries, pomegranate.

Did you know that strawberries and tomatoes are high in vitamin C. and that cherries are high in bioflavonoids, as are other berries? Cherries also contain rutin.

Tomatoes, a super food, contain melatonin and licopene which is one of the seven hundred carotenoids present in fruits and vegetables. Lycopene, an immune system booster, may be protective against prostate cancer, as well as being a potent antioxidant. Strawberries also contain lycopene.

Orange. Well, the most common thing we think of is an orange, a citric acid fruit that is very high in vitamin C, protective to the immune system. How about carrots and yams, which contain vitamin A and beta-carotene. Carrots are important for maintaining your eye sight.

Yellow. There are a number of vegetables that are yellow. Squash and beans are high in choline, essential in building the neurotransmitters (acetyl choline) that help keep our nervous system in tune, along with the B vitamins. How about bananas? Did you know bananas contain melatonin, which boosts our immune system and helps us sleep better? Onions contain selenium, which works together with the potent antioxidant, vitamin E.

Green. That's a big one. Green is the color of nature. It is the color of chlorophyll, the substance in green vegetables and plants and trees, which transforms sunlight into energy. Without chlorophyll and without the sunlight, we would not be able to live. The green fruits and vegetables are extremely important to us. Cruciferous vegetables, such as cabbage, kale, brussel sprouts and broccoli may even have anticancer effects. Broccoli, which you have heard a lot about, contains chromium, which helps maintain our insulin levels. Avocados contain magnesium, which is helpful in protecting the heart and boosting our memory. Magnesium even helps you sleep.

Dark green leafy vegetables are very high in carotene. In the previous chapter, I had a whole section on beta-carotene and its potent antioxidant properties. Dark green vegetables also contain a lot of vitamin E, as well as vitamin K, which is essential for normal blood clotting.

How about rutin, which is found in green peppers, as well as under the skins of citrus fruits, and as noted above in cherries? It is a bioflavonoid, which may be essential in suppressing tumors of the colon and helps fight increased cholesterol. It even helps in the absorption of vitamin C.

There are too many health benefits from all the greens to mention in this book, but some of the important greens are cucumbers, collard greens, Brussels sprouts, broccoli, cabbage (cabbage has been used as an anti-cancer and diet food), lettuces, spinach, kale, turnip greens and collards.

Blue. There are a number of fruits and even vegetables that have a blue color from blueberries to squashes. Blueberries are very potent anti-oxidants and are considered a super-food. How about the purple cabbage, which is loaded with nutrients. Blue-green algae is a popular supplement for detoxification programs. It is a potent antioxidant and anti-inflammatory agent.

As you can see from the examples given, the colors are important. Not only do they have medicinal and preventative health properties, they are also essential sources of organic minerals, vitamins, and enzymes, such as papain, which is in papaya. Papain is essential in the digestion of proteins and has been prescribed in Germany for years to aid in digestion and heartburn after big meals.

Did you know that papaya and pineapple also contain bromelain, which reduces inflammation, enhances immune function, and fights allergies and other inflammatory immune diseases?

Bromelain is essential in the digestion of starches and has been used as an anti-inflammatory agent. It is thought to reduce chronic inflammation, such as in arthritis and blood vessels (that can develop fatty deposits). So, maybe you should eat papaya and pineapple whenever you get a chance.

The rainbow foods, as I call them, are a good way for you to pick fruits and vegetables. Salmon, an excellent protein source high in Omega-3 fatty acids (which fight arteriosclerosis), is also red.

When you go shopping, just remember, the brighter the color, the better it is for you.

Eat fresh colors and you will be healthy, but make sure this stuff is not sprayed, and wash it thoroughly when you get home. You don't know what they've put on it to maintain its color. Sometimes producers spray, or gas, these vegetables and fruits to maintain their color so they'll have a longer shelf life. Just one more trick the food industry uses that may destroy the nutritional benefits of what we eat. (I've heard some horror stories about what grocers used to do, years ago, to keep old ground beef looking red.)

Let's get into even more specific anti-aging foods. It is impossible to cover the nutritional value of every single food. If you are interested, I recommend you go to the library and get college textbooks on nutrition, primarily from the dietetic point of view. Specific nutrition books will break down every single food and every single vitamin that it contains. You can also use the USDA or NIH web sites for information.

There is a lot of confusion on the internet with snippets of data being thrown at you from all sides. It is best to look at published textbooks or research articles in well-known journals written by PhDs and other doctors that specialize in nutrition. Unless an article is peer reviewed, it does not stand the scrutiny of science. Anyone can say anything, and if it is repeated enough it becomes established truth without proof. Remember that researcher I went to see? While his research was referenced all over, when I went to see the proof, Puff, it had vanished and the article was retracted by the journal.

In the next section of this chapter, I will cover specific foods that I believe are beneficial in longevity and give you the rationale behind them.

This afternoon, as I was dictating the first edition of this chapter on a porch filled with radiant warm Florida sunshine, I snacked occasionally on a pear, banana, or apple, which kept my sugar at a constant level, also filling me with essential vitamins. For supper, which I just finished, I had the rainbow foods.

I had a delicious carrot salad mixed with oranges from our back yard for flavor, along with a little cinnamon. It was absolutely delicious, and as a bonus gave me a tremendous amount of vitamins. I also had artichoke leaves and hearts, which gave me the greens. For protein and grains, I had spaghetti, with the meatballs having multigrain bread fortified with bran in them. As you can see from the meat, I am not a vegetarian and occasionally eat red meat. However, my diet consists primarily of large quantities of fruits and vegetables, and I limit my consumption of lean beef.

For protein, we primarily use various beans, lentils, skinless chicken breasts and fish, of which I recommend salmon and other cold water fish the most. Sardines and herring have higher concentrations of omega 3 and 6 fatty acids in them.

We also make tofu shakes, veggie burgers, and quite a few fruit shakes made in our high-powered blender. I prefer whole food shakes compared to extracted juices because of the roughage and the added nutrients from the skins of fruits and vegetables. Many fruits have most of the vitamins in the skins.

While I am on this topic, I do want to mention that steaming is preferable to boiling, because when you boil something you lose most of the minerals through the boiled water. Lightly steaming vegetables preserves most of the nutrients. You can also use the waterless cookware that slowly cooks the vegetables with almost no water, maintaining all its nutrients. I do not recommend canned vegetables and fruits except in emergencies, because most of the nutrients are blanched out. However, canned tomatoes do retain many nutrients.

One of my active retired patients taught me how to get the most vitamins out of vegetables as easily as possible: buy flash-frozen multi-vegetables that you can microwave or steam lightly, getting just about all the nutrients that are in fresh vegetables. Since he is single, it is an easy way for him to get a large variety of all his vegetables fairly rapidly, and the blended variety makes it taste good. The less heat and the less water you use in preparing vegetables, the more nutrients are preserved.

Through his ingenuity, he found a practical, useful solution to keep himself healthy. By the way, he is eighty years old, walks over a thousand miles a year and dances a couple of times a week. A clever man.

Bran

I feel bran is an important aspect of the longevity program because it keeps things moving in your gut. It is a great source of roughage and, believe it or not, it is non-caloric fiber containing vitamins such as riboflavin, thiamin, pantothenic acid, B1, B6, and niacin.

Bran is not the grain itself, but the coating of the seeds of grain, the shells of the seeds, such as in oats or wheat. It has been proven to relieve constipation, prevent diverticulitis, and has been known to stabilize cholesterol levels and decrease blood sugars for diabetics. But, the thing I like most about it is its propulsive effects. Food has to pass through your system and not hang around too much. If it hangs around a great deal, it promotes putrefaction and causes all kinds of intestinal problems, which can lead to colon cancer. By maintaining regular bowel movements with good consistency, and decreasing your blood sugar and cholesterol levels, you are getting a healthy aging nutritional effect.

While we are on that subject, don't forget to get your colonoscopy. A doctor friend of mine had to talk me into having mine done. I had mine without anesthesia, and slight discomfort, but I enjoyed watching my own anatomy on the monitor and those "cool" microvilli that do all of the nutrient absorption. Colon cancer is one of the most preventable cancers that we have. The polyps can be excised before they become cancerous.

Another grain that is beneficial is oats or oatmeal, which is also high in B vitamins, vitamin E, and various minerals, including iron.

Additionally, oatmeal contains protein and very high concentrations of soluble fiber, which also assists in lowering your cholesterol.

While working on the final edit of this book at beautiful Glacier National Park in Montana, I met a young couple riding bicycles loaded with gear. They had ridden nearly 5,000 miles and told me that their daily breakfast was oatmeal. So, here you have a couple of good foodstuffs you can have for breakfast: oatmeal and bran.

Cranberries

For your daily beverages, it is far better to have a mixture of a juice, such as cranberry juice and water, than any soft drinks or sugar drinks. I like cranberries as an anti-aging juice because it helps prevent urinary tract infections, which are quite common in the elderly. If these things are not prevented, you can become very ill and develop chronic septicemia, which can eventually lead to your death.

Cranberry juice's effectiveness against bladder and urinary tract infections is probably because it inhibits the growth of the bacteria in the uterine lining. Cranberry juice also helps lower blood pressure in animals.

One thing I like about having some cranberry juice in water is that it makes water, that I recommend drinking in large quantities, taste better. By protecting you from common infections of the urinary tract, you preserve your kidneys which filter the waste out of your system.

Garlic

I mentioned garlic earlier, but I think it is so important a longevity herb that I'll mention it again. Garlic needs to be a regular part of your anti-aging diet. Not only is freshly crushed (not dried) garlic antifungal, antibacterial, and antiviral, it may also protect you against liver damage and lower your serum cholesterol and triglyceride levels and protect your heart. Newest scientific research, published in the *Journal of Agricultural and Food Chemistry*, confirmed garlic's cardio protective effect by its release of small quantities of hydrogen sulfide gas. This process reduces heart damage developed from the lack of oxygen.

Garlic has also been shown to decrease platelet clotting, thereby thinning your blood and reducing your risk of clot-induced strokes. Have you ever wondered why the Mediterranean inhabitants have a low incidence of cardiovascular diseases? One of the reasons is their high consumption of garlic, and the other is consumption of olive oil.

Did you know that along with onions and chives, garlic boosts immunity? It helps fight infections and prevents cancers. It also helps neutralize toxins and free radicals. Some people also use it as an anti-stress agent.

The medicinal use of garlic goes as far as 6,000 years ago. It was used in several powerful countries, such as ancient Egypt, Rome and Greece. Hippocrates, the Greek Father of Medicine, recommended it as an antibiotic for infections. It was also used during the plague in France as a preventative agent.

In 1858, Louis Pasteur, the famous French microbiologist, was able to kill bacteria grown in a dish with garlic juice and reported on it in the medical literature.

The stories about garlic go on and on. As unpleasant as it may taste to some people, I personally like to take it on a regular basis as part of my longevity program. My grandmother in Poland, and my aunt that is a pharmacist in Germany, both used and recommended it for colds. My uncle used it for circulation and general health. Fresh, crushed, uncooked garlic is the best form to eat it, since crushing releases its enzymes. I like it on toast with tomatoes and oregano or chives for a pleasant sandwich. Aged garlic supplements are probably second best.

Soybeans

Soybeans are probably the most versatile, beneficial product you can have for health preservation and life extension.

Soy products, a great substitute for animal protein, should definitely be on your food list. You can buy it readily as protein powder or as a gelatinous substance known as tofu, which you can fry or mix with fruits, ice, and honey and make delicious shakes. The isoflavones in soy products lower the bad cholesterol (LDL), as well as triglycerides, and help raise the HDL portion of cholesterol, which is the good cholesterol.

The genistein portion of the isoflavones in soy has potent anti-cancer effects on laboratory animals. Besides that, the isoflavones in soybeans, which are glycetein, daidzein, and genistein, seem to work as weak estrogens in the body and are a great adjunct to any type of natural hormone replacement. Soybeans also contain phytates, which are active antioxidants and free radical scavengers.

In societies where diets are rich with soy products, there is a lowered incidence of all types of cancers. Soy is a complete protein just like meat, and contains all the essential amino acids, making it an excellent meat protein substitute. We use it in our soy veggie burgers, which taste almost exactly like regular hamburgers. It's amazing.

You can also try tempeh, which is a soy product that is fermented and has the consistency of meat, making it an excellent additive for casseroles or other dishes in which you would use ground beef.

Regular soy milk is all right, but it is a taste you have to get used to. You can, however, purchase chocolate and vanilla flavored soy milk which is absolutely delicious. Go ahead and try it. I have also used almond milk on my cereal and in coffee.

From replacing estrogen levels in post-menopausal women to reducing cholesterol, to its anti-cancer effects, soy has several benefits and can be a perfect substitute for meat. You may consider it as part of your longevity diet program. I recommend soy products routinely for my patients, especially those who are anemic and need higher protein intake to build up red blood cells, as well as muscles. My favorite soy products are tofu mixed in a fruit shake and soy powders.

For women, the phytoestrogenetic activity of soy products may protect them against the risks of developing cancers due to high estrogen levels, such as breast cancer and uterine cancer, as well as benign breast cysts. You see, the phytoestrogens from soy act like estrogens by occupying estrogen receptors and, therefore, they help regulate the estrogen level in a woman's body, having a gentle, protective effect. In the Far East, women take as much as 100 to 200 mg of isoflavones a day. As we all know, they have a very, very low incidence of breast cancer compared to women in the United States. However, when they move to the United States and start adapting to our diet, the breast cancer rate increases dramatically. Phytoestrogens are also found in nuts, seeds, whole grains, and beans.

Genistein, a potent phytoestrogen found in soy, is also available in capsule form and is generally taken in quantities of 80 mg a day or less. However, I feel that the total soy product is more beneficial than just an isolated component.

As you can tell from my discussion of soy, there are not enough good things that I can say about it. It is such a valuable food source that it should be a component of your anti-aging food program. For what it's worth, a good PhD friend of mine who is a vegetarian and is often mistaken as a 30-year-old despite his actual age of 59.

Oils

Our bodies need oils, and simultaneously essential fatty acids, but it is the type of oil we consume that is extremely important in relation to how our body metabolizes and uses it as an energy source. Essential fatty acids, such as alpha-linolenic acid and gamma-linolenic acid, the highest concentrations of which are found in flax seed oil, are essential. Other sources are sesame seeds, walnuts, pumpkin seeds, and soybeans.

Returning to the rainbow colors for a moment, dark green leafy vegetables also contain essential fatty acids, however, not as high a concentration as flax seed oil. You can also get essential fatty acids in borage oil.

These products need to be refrigerated and they do have an oily smell to them. You may want to take them in a capsular form of up to 1,000 to 5,000 mg twice a day.

Why are these good fats so important? Because they are essential fats, unlike the unhealthy bad fats. The transfats are found in high temperature cooking processes and the saturated fats are found in meat and dairy products. Those are called "vascular cloggers."

Unsaturated fats are vegetable oils, which include soy oil, sunflower oil, olive oil, safflower oil, and oils found in grains, seeds, nuts, and legumes.

So, why take essential fatty acids? Well, essential fatty acids have been declining in our diet over the past seventy-five years and a lack of essential fatty acids in our diet can be a contributing factor to a host of health problems ranging from inflammatory disorders to heart problems to arthritis. These essential fatty acids are nutrients, just like the minerals and vitamins we ingest, are important in maintaining life itself. The Mediterranean diet is considered one of the healthiest because it has unsaturated fats in it along with fruits and vegetables.

Essential fatty acids are used to manufacture cell membranes, which act as coverings for our cells and keep them from falling apart. The stronger the covering, the more impenetrable it is to invading organisms. These essential fatty acids are also important in the manufacture of prostaglandins, which act like hormones in your body, or like super enzymes, and help regulate important functions, such as fertility, conception, blood pressure, heart rate, blood clotting, pressure and inflammation on the eyes, joints and ears. As well, they affect the immune system and the nervous system, such as thinking, mood, and automatic reactions, as in the fight/flight mechanisms.

They also affect the skin moisture, healing properties, and secretions from various glands. Additionally, they influence kidney functions, heart functions, temperature regulation, fat deposits, appetite, sensitivity to cold, and various tumors and the spread of tumors. In other words, they concern every aspect of our body. That's why those essential fatty acids are essential.

Did you know that prostaglandins also regulate your inflammatory process? Inflammation is important because if you have an infective agent, you need the inflammatory process to help ward off and fight that agent. The inflammatory reaction is a healing process. The prostaglandins keep things in check, in a way, and keep the inflammation from becoming too large and devouring your whole body.

Prostaglandins work in pairs. One set of prostaglandins, which comes basically from arachidonic acid, is an essential fatty acid available in most diets. The other part of the prostaglandins comes from the alpha-linoleic acid and the gamma-linoleic acid, which are in short supply in our diet. Together they suppress the inflammatory response, keeping the inflammation in check. If you don't have enough of the essential fatty acids, you may have an inflammation that goes out of control, such as an allergic reaction.

As you can see, essential fatty acids are a very important component of your immune system and help trigger a variety of important functions in your body. From clot formation, allergic reaction, tissue swelling, hormone production and smooth muscle tone, these essential fatty acids are a vital part of your well-being.

Did you know they use prostaglandins to induce labor in childbirth? That's how important these hormone-like substances are, and they are derived from these essential fatty acids, which you must have in your diet and should be an important component of your longevity program.

Studies have shown that women consuming high concentrations of essential fatty acids have lower cancer rates, including breast cancer.

Did you know that they even regulate stomach secretions? You need enough acid secretion in your stomach to digest your foods. If you don't digest food properly, you won't get all the nutrients from it. Sometimes acidic foods, such as pickle juice, helps with digestion. My 83-year-old sister told me to drink pickle juice after eating because it's good for the digestion. It also may help with indigestion if you ate too much food.

So, take your essential fatty acids in the form of extra supplementation for a well-rounded longevity dietary program. You can take them in capsules or you can take the oils and put them on salads. Either way is fine. The most important thing is to supplement them externally since your diet is deficient in them.

There are two essential fatty acid families, the Omega-6 and the Omega-3 fatty acids. In more detail, the Omega-6 family includes linoleic acid, gamma-linolenic acid, and arachidonic acid. The Omega-3 family consists of alphalinolenic acid, eicosapentaenoic acid, and docosahexaenoic acid. All of these are essential fatty acids, which are broken down into the two families, with the Omega-3 family being especially cardio-protective.

Omega-3 fatty acids have received a lot of attention recently for being cardio-protective and studies have shown them to reduce LDL cholesterol, the bad cholesterol, as well as triglyceride levels. These Omega-3 fatty acids have also been shown to have antihypertensive effects on patients.

There have also been reports of improvement in people with rheumatoid arthritis after taking Omega-3 fatty acids. Sources of Omega-3 fatty acids include linseed oil, evening primrose oil, as well as flax seed oil. One of the most common sources are fish oils from oily fish, such as salmon, cod, mackerel, herring, and sardines. I give my patients neutral-tasting cod liver oil, which has a slight lemon flavor and contains very high concentrations of eicosapentaenoic acid and docosahexaenoic acid, as a protection for their cardiovascular systems.

There is a debate about consuming large quantities of fish to get your Omega-3 fatty acids because fish are now being constantly exposed to toxins, especially in coastal areas. Therefore, you need to stick to cold water fish species, such as salmon, tuna, cod, mackerel, and haddock, as well as herring, and avoid fish from industrialized or polluted coastal waters, which may have high concentrations of contaminants. Besides, you can get your Omega-3 fatty acids from flax seed oil and soy oil, as well as from vegetables and beans.

If you think you are getting protection by ordering a deep-fried fish burger as a fast food, think again. The deep-frying of the fish destroys the Omega-3 fatty acids and the high temperature of the grease causes trans-fatty acids, which clog up arteries with free radicals, and which will then increase your aging process. Do yourself a big favor: stick to the cold water fish, such as salmon, or take a good-tasting cod liver oil.

Omega-3 fatty acid products, as well as essential fatty acid products, can be found at our web site at *happylifehealthyaging.com* or you may visit your local health food store to see what is available. However, if you get cod liver oil, taste is always important. Make sure you get an oil that tastes neutral or has no flavor whatsoever, because if it doesn't taste good, you aren't going to take it. It took me a long time to find a product that actually tasted good and that patients would take without complaining.

Let's review the type of oils you should avoid and the type of oils you should take:

Avoid saturated fats, which are common in foods such as sausage, bacon, and chicken skins. It's the stuff that burns on the barbecue grill.

When eating animal protein, avoid the fat and get as lean a portion as possible.

Absolutely do not deep-fry anything. Although you need the oils this is not the way to get them.

You want to use unsaturated oils, which come from vegetable sources. You also need essential fatty acids, which come from flax seed oil and other oils.

For cardiac protection, stick to the Omega-3 fatty acids.

The best source of vegetable protein is soy protein, which also contains isoflavones and has a myriad of beneficial health effects.

Grains, Breads, and Starches

Just like good cholesterol and bad cholesterol, there are good grains and bad grains.

What are the bad grains? Anything bleached and highly processed, such as white bread or white rice.

What are the good grains? Anything that is whole and left alone as it is in nature and contains large quantities of fiber and complex carbohydrates, as well as vitamins and minerals.

Did you know that whole rye bread contains more minerals, vitamins, and protein than whole wheat bread? I remember eating whole rye bread growing up as a child in Europe. It was completely different from the mushy stuff you buy in the grocery store today. What we are buying now is processed rye bread. Read the ingredients, you may be surprised to see what it actually contains.

Whole rye bread has much more protein, phosphorus, calcium, iron, thiamin, niacin, and other vitamins and minerals than processed rye bread. As mentioned previously, it is more nutritious than whole wheat bread. Try to get the whole rye kernel rather than the processed rye kernel, and the taste will be amazing.

Rice is a common food used throughout the world. Did you know that one pound of white rice contains four times the food energy as the same weight of potatoes? The problem with white rice is that the husk, bran, and germ are removed, leaving a product that is mostly starch.

The best form of rice is brown rice, which also contains the bran and the germ component of it, and is rich in B vitamins and iron.

Wheat is probably the most common grain used in the United States. The problem with it, again, is that over the years it has been genetically modified and refined. People have become allergic to it and consequently require gluten free diets.

Therefore, it is good to alter the grains in your diet.

Corn is a potent nutrient in our diet and is grown extensively throughout the world. It contains complex carbohydrates and essential vitamins, such as riboflavin and niacin. However, it lacks two essential amino acids, lysine and tryptophan. These amino acids need to be supplemented from other sources. Basically, pure corn on the cob is a good form of carbohydrate starch. Surprisingly enough, corn on the cob is also a low calorie food.

Corn syrup is also used as a sweetener in many processed foods. If you read the labels almost everything has corn syrup as a sweetener in it. Ever wonder why there is such a high incidence of diabetes, and now juvenile diabetes in young children? Carbohydrates lead to obesity and sugar leads to obesity and we consume much too much of both, willingly or unwillingly.

Potatoes are an excellent low-calorie source of food. They are loaded with carbohydrates and, if you eat the skin, you will get a large dose of vitamins, as well as protein. In Europe, the potato is a mainstay of essential minerals and vitamins.

I remember hearing stories where during World War II the prisoners in the gulags of Russia were given potato peels, while the guards ate the potatoes. In the end, the prisoners were eating a healthier meal than the guards, allowing them to survive the cold bitter winters of Siberia and to make it home after the war.

The only thing you have to remember about potatoes, to get the added nutrition you need, is to keep the skin on and don't add fat. Eat potatoes in moderation since they are high in carbohydrates and convert to blood sugar easily. Sweet Potatoes are a good alternative.

A good example of a protective food is naturally fermented cabbage.

In 2005, researchers in Poland discovered that female Polish immigrants to the USA were experiencing a breast cancer rate three times higher than those living in Poland. They knew that the cause had to be environmental. After careful observation of the polish women living in Detroit and Chicago, they noted that in Poland the women were consuming 30 pounds of natural lacto-fermented sauerkraut per year while in the USA they only ate 10 lbs. The natural fermentation process increases the bioavailability of nutrients in the cabbage which act as a protective mechanism against breast cancer.

Sauerkraut contains high levels of glucosinolates which, laboratory studies have found to contain anti-cancer properties, as observed in the research on immigrant polish women. Glucosinolates may protect against DNA damage and restrict cancer cell growth. Research is being conducted at the University of New Mexico to determine how that process works. Dorothy Rybaczyk-Pathak from the University of New Mexico and scientists at Michigan State University and the National Food and Nutrition Institute of Warsaw, Poland, concluded that "Women who ate at least three servings a week of raw, or short-cooked cabbage and sauerkraut, had a significantly reduced breast cancer risk compared with those who only ate one serving per week."

It is important that the sauerkraut be naturally fermented and not processed with chemicals. You can find natural sauerkraut in the refrigerated sections of your grocery store. The leuconostoc and lactobacillus bacteria that ferment the sauerkraut actually live on the leaves. All you need is shredded cabbage, salt and an airtight container.

Another food with similar gut health qualities is Kimchi, the Korean version of sauerkraut. Kimchi is a naturally fermented blend of vegetables usually containing cabbage, salt, garlic, onions, red peppers, ginger, celery, carrots or other vegetables.

Both cabbage and sauerkraut help to restore our gut flora that is often decimated by antibiotics.

The newest buzzword in biochemical research is our "human microbiome." The human microbiome is a diverse world of microorganisms that inhabit our bodies and promote our health. The US National Institute of Health is just now starting to study which microorganisms are associated with both healthy and unhealthy humans. The larger the diversity of our gut flora, the healthier we humans may be.

It turns out that our gut environment, as shown through the sauerkraut observations, is far more important than doctors ever thought. If they knew how important our gut flora is for health, they would not have prescribed antibiotics for every sniffle. Antibiotics not only kill the bad bacteria but also the good bacteria in our gut that keep us healthy. Restoring a diverse gut flora through probiotics is extremely important for our overall health.

Fermented sauerkraut, kimchi, various yogurt strains, sour milk, kefir and other probiotic strains will go a long way towards restoring your gut flora to a healthier environment.

A PhD friend of mine had a visiting professor from the Czech Republic go to a doctor in the USA for a bad flu. After the doctor gave her a prescription for antibiotics he sent her on her way. Before leaving, the professor asked, "What are you going to give me as a probiotic?" The US doctor stood dumbfounded. She had to explain that in Europe when a doctor gives you an antibiotic he will also give you a probiotic to restore your natural gut flora. You take the antibiotic first for 10 days and then take the probiotic so that you have biodiversity in your gut and the bad bacteria, such as clostridium difficile (C. Diff.), doesn't overgrow in your gut and kill you.

This overgrowth happened to a cousin of mine after cardiac surgery in Jacksonville, Florida. He was discharged from the hospital and in three days readmitted because of declining health. By the time they figured out what was wrong, C. Diff. had overgrown in his entire gut and dispersed into his bloodstream, killing him in a few days. The prophylactic antibiotics he had taken before surgery had killed the good gut bacteria that would have kept the C. Diff in balance, but did not kill all the C. Diff. After surgery the C. Diff multiplied unopposed by other organisms in the gut and eventually killed him.

There is a good reason why the USA is ranked 37[h] in overall health out of 181 countries by the World Health Organization (WHO) despite the amount of money we put into our health care. Even though we are spending the highest percentage of our GDP on health care, it appears that other countries are practicing better preventive medicine, and not just focusing on high ticket items that pay the most profit. France provides the overall best health care followed by Italy, Spain, Oman, Australia and Japan.

Since the first edition of this book came out a great deal of interest on gut bacterial flora composition (microbiome or biome) has developed in the microbiological science world. It is estimated that the human mouth may have more than 700 distinct organisms. The human gut has a lot more. Older estimates of the number of distinct gut organisms were in the 500 – 1500 range. This number was determined by growing bacteria in petri dishes that only showed the most common organisms. Newer studies at Stanford University done by the David Relman group, used pyrosequencing through DNA tags. Their research upped that distinct organism number in your gut to 5,600. That's a lot of different organisms. They all work together as a symbiotic symphony eating up our digested food, producing vitamins, fine tuning our immune system and keeping the bad bacteria in check.

It appears that at least two of the bacteria in your gut produce a neurotransmitter called GABA. Behavioral conditions such as mood and autism have been correlated with the composition of the gut bacteria microbiome. The type of bacteria in your gut may make a difference in how you feel. The vagus nerve runs directly from your brain to your gut and can theoretically relay messages from your gut bacteria to your brain. These messages could be a crosstalk network signaling your brain to form certain chemicals that influence a host of physiological function in your body, from how you feel to the metabolism of your food and nutrient absorption.

There is an epiphany going on in endocrinology right now. Endocrinology used to be simply associated with the secretory organs that produced all kinds of hormones, such as testosterone, estrogen, growth hormone and so on. Now, it appears that almost all cells in the body talk to one another, including all those little bugs that live in your gut! Not to get too carried away, but your gut microbiome is extremely important to your overall health and healthy aging. So, make sure that you have a diverse blend of bacteria living inside you, cheering you on to live longer.

For the newest updates on gut microflora research, and how to replenish your gut bacteria biodiversity, refer to our web site *www.happylifehealthyaging.com.*

What should you eat? The US government department of health, *www.health.gov/ dietary guidelines*, officially released their new guidelines in 2016 which took a reverse course from its previous guidelines. Now it is acceptable to have cholesterol from eggs.

Saturated fats found in fatty meats, and high-fat dairy products, increase blood cholesterol more than dietary cholesterol in eggs does.

The sugars are the culprit. No more than 10 percent of your calories should be from sugars. Sugars are in much of the processed foods, such as sauces, relishes, ketchup and the dressings we eat. Just one can of soda will max out your sugar limit of 50 grams/day. If you add breads and cookies to that, you are way over the limit. Unfortunately, this happens more often than not in America, and is the stem of many health issues. The pounds start piling up around your hips, your belly and inside your abdomen.

I know a lady that was thin her whole life until after retiring when she took up baking breads and cookies. Guess what happened? Forty lbs. later she had to give all of her beautiful clothes away because "they shrunk." Carbohydrates will put on pounds and increase your blood sugar and blood pressure faster than a speeding bullet.

The solution is simple. Do not keep carbohydrate foods in the house. That means pastries, cookies, donuts, white bread, crackers and snack foods. You can have high density multigrain bread in your freezer to make toast each day, but eating a lot of bread piles on the carbs, which piles on the fat, just as sugars do. Whole grains are good for you in cereals but don't forget to sprinkle flax seed on top of them for essential fatty acids.

Less meat, especially processed meat, is beneficial for your cardiovascular health. Fish continue to be highly recommended for their omega 3, 6 fatty acids since they are cardio protective. The cold water fatty fish along with sardines, herring and wild salmon are loaded with those protective fatty acids.

How about salt? Most of us eat way too much salt. Salt stresses your cardiovascular system and can lead to high blood pressure. The new guidelines recommend no more than a teaspoon per day about 2300 milligrams, but for better heart protection stick to less than three quarters of a teaspoon, about 1500 milligrams. Read the labels for salt content and try to purchase less salty foods. You can also use a variety of spices for flavoring food rather than salt.

The guidelines also strongly emphasize 2.5 cups of mixed vegetables along with 2 cups of fruits. Just remember the rainbow colored foods that I talked about and you will do fine. Wine is good, and the Mediterranean diet seems to be the healthiest. It's nice to see that the new guidelines are more in line with what I talked about in 2000.

Juices

There are a large variety of juices used for longevity benefits and health promotion. The most common vitamin-rich juices that we are familiar with are citric juices, such as grapefruit and orange. I have previously mentioned the benefits of cranberry juice. People are even consuming aloe vera juice for its anti-inflammatory protective effects, both for your digestive system and applying it externally on sun burns.

I have patients who attribute their strength and stamina in old age to beet juice. Others espouse the benefits of a Tahitian drink from the Noni plant. Carrot, spinach, cucumber, cabbage, broccoli and tomato juice are also favorites either alone or in combinations.

Any fruit or vegetable can be turned into a drink. From blueberries to cherries to limes to mulberries, to lemons, raspberries, prunes, pineapple, and watermelon. By the way, pure watermelon juice is very good tasting. It is an excellent thirst-quencher in the summer time and is loaded with vitamins.

Most of us drink orange juice, but there are many other juices and nectars available, as well, that taste fantastic and are healthy. The only problem is you have to drink pure juice, not canned juices or juice drinks, which contain high concentrations of corn syrup or fruit sweetener. The sweeteners are essentially sugar that is converted to fat in your body, unless you burn it up as you drink while exercising.

If you are buying fruit juice, always buy pure fruit juice without any additives or sweeteners. The best option, however, is to get fresh fruit and make your own fruit juice so that you know what you're getting.

Fruit juice is a good way of getting many vitamins because they are so concentrated. Whole fruit juices are even better because they also contain the skin and the pulp of the fruit, giving you more nutrient vitamins and minerals than you would get from extracted juices. As well, they are a great source of roughage, which your body needs for a longevity program. The colored skin of the fruit or vegetables, as previously mentioned, is where most of the vitamins are.

Sometimes it may be more practical to drink juice instead of eating the food itself. For example, carrot juice can be very filling and easier to consume than chopped up carrots that you can choke on. You get a lot more concentrated nutrition from the carrot juice itself.

A popular healthy drink is also a green drink made from a variety of green vegetables including cabbage, sweetened with carrots or beets. For those of you without teeth, or with poor-quality dentures, whole food juicing is definitely the way to go to get all your nutrients from fruits and vegetables. Get a juicing cookbook that will describe tasty combinations. Whole juices are generally better than extracted juices because they contain pulp which is roughage with vitamins.

Remember, five servings of fruits and vegetables a day are recommended and will give you large quantities of B6 and folic acid. Folic acid is shown to reduce heart disease through various studies. Since heart disease is a major factor in early death, increasing your quantities of fruits and vegetables will help to reduce your chance of dying early. Heart disease accounts for nearly 610,000 deaths per year, or one quarter of all deaths in the US. You may also reduce your chance of dying early from cancer because of the phyto-chemicals that are protecting your immune system. Not to mention the fact that you are strengthening the building blocks of your bones, connective tissues, organs, brain, and skin, as well as increasing your antioxidant protection, and, in turn keeping you healthy and vigorous.

I hope this chapter on fruits, vegetables and dietary choices nudged you towards making wiser choices in what you eat. It is good to know why you are doing something instead of just taking some magic pill that you know nothing about. Every human body is slightly different. This is the only body that we have, so we had better make sure we give it the best building blocks possible in order for it to grow healthy and repair itself when things go wrong. Don't skimp on high quality organically grown food. It's like an investment in the best building materials for your home.

CHAPTER 9

The Healthy Mind, Active, Happy,

And Stress-Free

It is 5 o'clock in the morning. My mind is working at a feverish pace to come up with a proper title for this chapter. I had numerous ones written down, but few of them had the spirit of what I am about to tell you. Finding the right words is oftentimes more difficult than you think.

Do you remember how difficult it was to tell someone for the first time that you loved him or her? You were sweating bullets, weren't you? How would that person react? Were you going to be accepted? After all, you were totally vulnerable, weren't you?

But your mind and spirit were ready for a new experience. You were willing to risk it for a greater benefit. The benefit of total ecstasy and invulnerability, to be on Cloud Nine where nothing else mattered except you and your partner. The feeling of love is a very powerful emotion. It can move mountains, part the sea, and make you feel as if you are invincible.

I can still remember going to church while in middle school, many years ago, and speaking to a clergyman. I asked him what made people happy. His response was, "In order to be happy in life, you have to give more than you get." For a twelve-year-old, that concept was rather difficult to comprehend. I thought and thought and thought about it.

How could you survive if you gave more than you got? It was impossible to do that. You'd end up with a negative balance of whatever you had. You'd be in the hole.

After a while, I figured it out, and guess what.

"The more you give, the more you get."

"Whatever good deeds you do come back to you a thousand fold."

"What goes around comes around."

You must have heard these statements throughout your life. Have you ever put any thought to them? Let me tell you one thing. People who follow those rules are happy, alert, and stress-free into very old age.

There is a power in the universe that keeps track of things. It keeps track of your good thoughts and your bad thoughts, your good and bad intentions. It is a life force of energy and creativity and your goodness towards humanity.

My mother had a powerful life force. She was kind to others and made people feel good. She was always cheerful. I almost never heard her complain. She was a true friend and a vibrant soul. I have never seen anyone else have as many true friends as she did.

She had young friends and old. Former bosses were friends. College students were friends. She had friends of different religions. As a matter of fact, after she died, she was baptized again, in a completely different religion, because they thought so highly of her that they wanted to make sure she went to heaven. Now those are true friends, people who worry about your soul even after you're dead.

She had a tremendous life force inside her, a spirit that influenced everyone for the better. I have pictures of her camping out in the gorgeous canyons and painted deserts of Utah, going on hiking trips with university students considerably younger than herself. She loved to sing, dance, have fun, get together with people, and volunteer her free time for whatever was needed. She made people feel good.

On lectures, at adult living facilities, I can always find people like her. They are the ones smiling, attentive, bright, bushy-tailed and cheery-eyed. They are interested in life. They have keen minds. They can follow my lectures and ask intelligent questions. They smile a lot. They make my trip to their retirement home worthwhile. These are people in their late eighties, nineties and even over a hundred.

We have many of these people around the St. Petersburg - Tampa Bay area because people love to come here to the warm climate to retire.

When I ask Activities Directors about them, they tell me these men and women have the best health and the least ailments. They inform me numerous times that those over a hundred are in a much better physical shape than some of those in their seventies who are always complaining, worrying, and predicting that bad things are going to happen. Believe it or not, bad things do happen to them.

Those with the greatest attitude towards life take things one day at a time, and they enjoy things fully. They always have. They live life and they know that they are living. Life is an adventure for them and they don't worry. As the song goes, "Don't worry, be happy."

Jessie, a spry 94 year old that I recently interviewed in Newfoundland told me "don't sweat the small stuff."

When I met this thin, attractive, well-dressed lady at the level one adult living facility that she lived in, I was impressed by the stacks of large print crossword puzzle books she had next to her rocking chair. She said "you've got to keep your mind going, because without your mind you have nothing."

She liked living there because of all the friends she had made. To her, having friends was very important.

Her husband was a fisherman and she would always help him out whenever he came home from a trip. As well, she would gather the firewood, chop it up herself, and do a lot of the physical work by herself because her husband was frequently gone cod fishing. They ate the food they grew or that was fished in the ocean. For entertainment she would get together with friends to socialize and have some tea and cakes.

During our conversation I asked her what she liked to do for fun. She stated that she liked to dance. Suddenly, a glimmer came into her eye as she reminisced about an old boyfriend from another town that used to take her dancing. She had lost contact with him as he had moved away, but she still talked about him fondly as if it were yesterday. Those passionate moments of dancing on the dance floor with a boyfriend seventy five years ago were as clear to her today as they were then.

What I noticed from this very alert 94-year-old lady was that she was actively participating in her longevity program. She used to walk a lot until she tripped and fell, breaking her hip, but she was still socially engaged. She realizes that in order to enjoy life at that age, she has to keep her mind stimulated by doing those crossword puzzles. She said that she didn't eat a lot, just enough to keep her going. Food wasn't a top priority in her life. Having friends, being active and staying mentally engaged had a higher priority. Jessie had inner happiness, peace of mind and a warm friendliness about her that everyone loved.

Inner happiness, kindness, peace of mind, and a strong desire to give of yourself are the most important longevity attributes that you can have.

By now you must be saying, "Oh how sweet, but where's the beef?" The "beef" is sandwiched inside your skull. It's all in your mind.

You have free will.

You can decide from this day forward that you will have a happy mind. You will turn your biggest adversity into your greatest asset by not letting it get the better of you. You will make lemonade out of lemons. You will make people feel wonderful around you and be happy that they are alive because of your presence. You are going to be a positive person, having as much fun as possible, while doing as much good as possible for the people around you, be it your spouse, your children, your neighbors, or people in your church, synagogue, or mosque, as well as for the animals and plants around you.

You will be kind to nature. Every little plant has sensation, which has been proven over and over again in numerous biological experiments. The plants for which you have happy thoughts grow well and thrive. The plants you don't admire and care for shrivel away and die, even though they get the same amount of sunlight, water, and nutrition.

Your thoughts influence everything around you. You possess the ability to change the way you think.

Did you know that when it became the first month of the year 2000, that is January of 2000, there were a large number of deaths in New York? I remember reading about it in the newspaper. They compared statistics about the death rate at the beginning of that year with other years. The reason the death toll was so high that January was because those people chose to live into the new millennium! They chose to live! Then, once they got there they said, okay, it's time to let go, and they passed on.

A friend of mine died recently. She was a realtor, a bubbly person. She waited until her relatives were there at her side. About ten minutes after the last one arrived, she died. My mother did the same thing. I flew back from Mexico City to be at her side, sitting next to her, holding her hand, and talking to her. Within six hours, she took her last breath and died, peacefully and happily.

Your mind controls your biological functions. You mind controls your hormone levels. Your mind controls your spirit. Your mind controls your anti-aging processes. "Smile and the whole world smiles with you. Cry and you cry alone." It is all in your mind.

By now, you must be saying, "Dr. Lenhart, this isn't a motivational book. This is a book about healthy aging." Guess what? Your mental attitude is one of the secrets to healthy aging. How sharp your mind is determines how well and how long you are going to live. It also determines your quality of life, and how happy you are.

If you're not happy, get out there and start doing volunteer work. Help people who are in need and you'll find out how lucky you truly are. Go out to the nursing homes, hospitals, and children's centers. Go to an animal shelter; even help a poor dog or cat find a new home. Help a child in need, become a big brother or big sister. Get involved, help out. By helping others you will be helping yourself, because your mind needs to be constantly stimulated in order to stay young.

The old theories about aging were that the mind, throughout its lifetime, slowly lost its brain cells and atrophied. If you look at an MRI or CT scan, taken of an older person, you will see a lot more fluid-filled spaces and less density in the brain matter. Everyone thought that was a natural progression in aging, until recently, when those old theories were re-evaluated. You see, most brains being studied had brain diseases such as senility and Alzheimer's disease. These findings did not include brains of active, mentally alert adults. They made assumptions that everyone's brains degenerated and atrophied. That assumption was wrong. How could Einstein be actively making new discoveries well into old age? How could Linus Pauling be running his research institute well into old age? These people stayed mentally alert and engaged. I met a social anthropology university professor recently at a folk festival who plans on working until he is eighty.

You want to hear another secret? The greater your education, either formal or self–taught, the greater become your chances of staying mentally alert through old age. As long as you are inquisitive about life, intelligence will stay with you. You are always stressing your neurons and forming new dendrites. You may be saying, "What are you talking about?" Let me backtrack.

Your brain has cells called nerve cells, which have stems attached to them. Those stems have very small branches coming off them, and those branches have even smaller branches coming off of them called dendrites. The more densely packed your dendrites are, those tiny little twigs coming off nerve cells, the greater your ability to make connections. The more education you have, the more you have proliferated those dendrites, the more variety of activities you have done and interests you have engaged in, the greater will be your cluster of dendritic connections.

One important thing, however, is that you need variety. When you get older, your dendritic thought patterns start to crystallize into one place. That means that whatever you've been doing all your life, you're still good at. For example, a great composer in his nineties will likely be a greater composer because of his wisdom, knowledge, and experience. However, other capabilities diminish. The composer will be good at composing and that's it. Other things are going to be lacking. Variety in activities, variety in living environments and variety in mental stimulation will keep your dendrites sprouting and keep you mentally alert.

A great musician can play music well into old age. Music is a mental stimulant and is very important in our anti-aging program. I believe it has something to do with the pleasure sensors in our brain. When you are constantly stimulating your pleasure sensors, your mind will be happy and continue to thrive.

Remember when I highlighted the Kids 'n Kubs, the St. Petersburg baseball team where the players were in their 80's? Because of their constant repetition of the sport, they crystallized those activities throughout their life and were able to perform them quite well into their old age. Unknowingly, they also improved their mind by physical activity. Through increased blood supply they kept their neurons stimulated.

Let's get into basic research. Studies on rats were created to determine how their brains reacted to different stimuli. Typically, rats were locked up in cages; let's call them condominiums. They would basically walk around inside their four walls (let's call it the living room, efficiency kitchen, and bedroom) and didn't do much else.

When these rats died, their brains were dissected and evaluated for dendritic density to determine how many nerve connectors they had. They found that over time, the number of nerve connectors diminished. Their brains got smaller. They were quite content to be in their rat condominium, within their four walls, not doing much of anything. They died with a smaller brain and that was it.

They took another group of rats and changed their environment. Every day they put them in a new and exciting environment, with different toys and new areas they could explore. They could also interact with other rats. "How ya doing this morning? Having fun exploring this environment? Isn't it a beautiful day? Look at this old sock and shoe we can get into."

They had a wonderful time. Then they were put back in their cages (condominiums). The next day, they were taken out again and put into a box in which all the furniture had been rearranged. Different toys were there for them to play with, so they had a stimulatingly new environment every time they got out of their condominium.

When it finally became time to see their maker, the rats' brains were sliced up. Guess what the researchers found? These rats had the brains of young rats, full of dendrites. They didn't age at all. They had anti-aging brains.

Mental stimulation caused them to stay young. They got out and they got involved. With a new challenge every day, the rats were mentally, aesthetically, physically, and socially stimulated. They got to meet each other, do things, interact, explore. They got out of their four-wall condominiums and explored the rest of the world.

Now, you may be saying to yourself, "Well, that makes sense, mental stimulation and new environment keeps them mentally alert. So where do those baseball players fit in?" That's what those researchers thought, although they were not dealing with baseball players, they were dealing with rats. They gave these little rats in the confined environment a gym. Every day those rats, instead of just sitting around in their cages looking at their four walls, were given a treadmill, which is that little wheel they run on. These rats got in there and started doing exercises. They ran that wheel in circles for hours, getting a good cardiovascular workout by the end.

When it was time for them to be sacrificed, their brains were, once more, sliced into little pieces, and guess what? They had an increased dendritic pattern and increased connectors in their brains. Their brains stayed young. The increased physical activity kept their minds young. Even though they didn't have as stimulating an environment as did the other rats, they were given increased exercise which was enough to increase the blood flow to the brain. Physical exercise also stimulates the nerve endings of the brain so that they don't atrophy.

There is less chance of atrophy when you are physically active. Maybe that explains the perfect shape, mentally and physically, of my elderly neighbor who walked several miles a day, although it probably didn't hurt that he was also writing poetry and trading stocks.

Pets also seem to make people younger. I remember seeing documentaries of people with amazing dogs and cats who took their pets to children's hospitals and nursing homes and where it made everyone perk up. They become alive, interactive, and they all loved to pet these animals. Even people in wheelchairs who are inanimate, just sitting there, all of a sudden become active and involved with these pets.

Pets, such as cats and dogs, seem to stimulate the brain and influence the pleasure sensors in our brains, aiding longevity. Sick children do better around these animals. Feeble, older adults respond and become younger again. There is a magic quality to pets that helps to keep us young in our old age.

If you have a dog, it makes you go out at least once a day for a walk, which you normally might not do. It makes you care for something, and a dog gives you a tremendous amount of love, affection and companionship. Cats are different creatures altogether. They give you a tremendous amount of company, love, and physical interaction through their mannerisms, various moods, and playfulness. They are also extremely easy pets to care for. I call them pocket pets.

All you have to give them is food, water, and a litter box, which you clean once a week. So, if you are active doing sports, going to the gym, doing all kinds of activity, you may want to consider a cat because they are a lot less work to care for. I had both and I'll tell you, the dogs were a lot more work.

You have to be very, very careful what kind of pet you choose because dogs and cats are a long term commitment. If you are very active and go away a lot on trips, having a dog that has to be walked twice a day can become expensive. You either have to kennel them or hire a dog sitter. Taking pets to hotels, restaurants and across international borders can be a problem also. So although these animals are beneficial towards longevity, there is also a responsibility to consider. Pet owners are limited in their freedom. You do not want to become a caregiver to a pet and limit your lifestyle during the years that you can still be very active traveling, enjoying the world. How are you going to take a 2 week or 2 month cruise? At an older age, when you don't do as much, pets may be a good choice for your lifestyle and companionship.

Let's get back to basic research. We're getting a little carried away here. By now, you must be following my train of thought and drawing conclusions of my analogies. Fine. But what's the best combination?

Let's backtrack a little. Earlier on, I mentioned a hormone called cortisol. It is a stress hormone released when the body and mind are under prolonged or tremendous stress. It is a destructive hormone. It ages you rapidly, destroys brain cells, and causes damage to your tissues. Have you ever seen anyone who has been on cortisone for any period of time? They puff up. Sometimes their bones get very frail and brittle and they break or degenerate. Other organ systems start to fail. Well, that's what stress does to you.

Stress increases the cortisol level, which destroys our bodies over time. Mental and emotional stress is a tremendous aging factor. It causes us to age prematurely and die early.

Since increased stress is health destroying, a reduction of stress must be an important component in your healthy aging program. Like Jessie said "don't sweat the small stuff."

The more of a stress-free environment you surround yourself with, the happier and healthier you will be. "But," you are saying, "Dr. Lenhart, you started out this chapter with the subject of love. What's love got to do with it?" The answer is, everything.

Love is the most potent emotion in the universe. The more you can be in the state of love, the happier and healthier your mind is going to be. It could be love for your spouse, love for your pet, love of your neighbor, love of the work that you do, love of a hobby or love of a sport. The more loves you can put together, the brighter your life is going to be.

Let's put things into perspective. A while back, I was lecturing to a local Optimist International Service Club. For their appreciation of my lecture on nutrition and chelation therapy, they gave me a plaque called The Optimist Creed, which reads:

Promise yourself to be strong, that nothing can disturb your peace of mind,

To talk health, happiness, and prosperity to every person you
    meet,

To make all your friends feel that there is something in them,

To look at the sunny side of everything and make your
    optimism come true,

To think only the best, to work only for the best, and expect
    only the best,

To be just as enthusiastic about the success of others as you are
    about your own,

To forget the mistakes of the past and press on to greater
    achievement of the future,

To wear a cheerful countenance at all times and give every
    living creature you meet a smile,

To give so much time to the improvement of yourself
    that you have no time to criticize others,

To be too large for worry, too noble for anger, too strong
    for fear, and too happy to permit the presence of
    trouble.

I thought that was a wonderful creed for the Optimists International Organization. It also reminds me of the quotation of Marjorie Hertz, the ninety-eight year old woman living in Naples, Florida, I previously mentioned. I recite it in my lectures to other doctors on physical activity and anti-aging. Remember her motto?

"Smile awhile and while you smile, another smiles, and soon there are miles and miles of smiles, and life's worthwhile because you smiled."

Aren't those two quotes wonderful? Just think, if you are always smiling to other people, you are creating good will and that smile gets carried on and on to other people and passes on good karma to the universe. Remember, what goes around comes around. It's going to come back to you many fold. It's going to make your life richer. It's going to reduce your aging process.

A smile can go a long way. Just remember, a smile is one of the best stress reducers out there.

Remember when I talked about how cortisol levels are related to stress and mental deterioration? You can avoid that by smiling. You can avoid that by not letting anything disturb you. You can avoid that by having peace of mind. You can avoid that by talking health, happiness, and prosperity to every person you meet.

In a previous chapter I mentioned a patient of mine who is a beautician at adult living facilities. When I questioned her about the young/old and the old/old, she stated without hesitation that the young/old, that is people in their nineties or older, are in better shape more often than people twenty years younger, because they have a much better attitude. They talk prosperity and health. They talk about happiness. They talk about the joy in life. They talk about doing things, being involved. They take one day at a time and live it to the fullest. Those who are always talking about their bad health, how rotten things are, how they are going to fall and break their hip, talking about the misery of others, and constantly complaining, believe it or not their predictions come true. Those people do die younger.

What your mind can perceive, it will achieve. If they perceive negative thoughts, emotions, and events, then the universe gives it to them. They develop poor health. They have all kinds of problems. Those who smile and talk health, prosperity, and joy generally avoid those problems because they have a great weapon in their healthy aging arsenal working for them, their mind and attitude.

You can improve your mind.

I remember seeing a story about an eighty-nine year old woman who got a degree from Harvard. It took her sixteen years to get, but she got it. Even at age eighty-nine, you can still sprout new dendrites by stimulating your mind. You don't have to forget where you left the keys or whom you talked to five minutes ago. You can stay mentally alert and sharp just by exercising your mind. It's a potent anti-aging tool. You exercise your mind by using it. If physical exercise increases the oxygenation to the brain, then mental exercise increases the proliferation of the brain.

A lot of people have great long-term memory and poor short-term memory when they get older. The long-term memory is sort of fixed in your hard drive, which is another part of your brain, and your short-term memory is in your RAM, which is the random access memory in your computer. You can increase your RAM by mental stimulation.

Old people oftentimes just love to talk about old events. Those events are impregnated in the hippocampus, a part of the brain that stores old data where you had emotional experiences and which the brain decided is important to keep. The short-term memory in the cortex is very fluid. It comes and goes. It decreases with age because it's not used. It is not continuously stimulated.

So, what is your job? Your job is to increase the RAM in your mind computer, constantly forcing it to be upgraded. You do that by mental enhancements such as mind games. Remember the Mankato study on nuns who donated their brains to science. In an autopsy it was found they had the brains of young people, even though they were ninety years old, because they were playing mind games continuously. I remember watching a show of an old chess champion who was very competitive, even in his old age, because he was constantly stimulating his mind trying to outwit his opponents. Card games are also good, as are complex jigsaw puzzles, which give you spatial orientation.

Expert witnesses for courtroom cases may be specialists who do one thing only, and study one thing only, instead of someone with a varied knowledge base of information. That's great for the courtroom, but that single focus knowledge doesn't do much to keep you young and other areas of your brain will shrivel up.

The more you study, the more things you do, the younger your mind will be. You have a quest for knowledge. You enjoy variety. You have an anti-aging mind. When you get older, you will be as sharp as a tack. As long as you keep feeding that mind new information, it will continue to grow. Your mental acuity will not deteriorate. Learning new things on a variety of subjects will keep your mind constantly stimulated and will increase the RAM in your memory circuits. The cortex of your brain will be forced into action. When that happens, your overall memory will improve. Your short-term retention will improve. You will be less forgetful and able to multitask again.

I noticed that when my chelation patients added vitamins to their IV therapy, their short term memory improved. They didn't have to write as many notes. Overall, they were mentally more competent. I believe that result is primarily due to increased circulation to the brain and increased mental stimulation. Exercising alone will increase endorphins, make you feel better, and increase the oxygenation to the brain, giving you greater capacity. That increased capacity has to be enhanced by mental stimulation, through learning new things.

Go back in your life and think of all the things you have ever been interested in. Make a list. Be creative. Go back to your early childhood. What turned you on? What did you like? Then go decade by decade. Try to find milestones in your life.

People think life is a series of milestones in which they put flags that they can remember things by. I go by dates as to how old I was in a certain year. It's easy for me since I was born in an even-numbered year, I can figure out how old I was when something was happening in my life. So, when they mention a certain event in history, I can recall that I was that age and doing these kind of things at that age. It gives me a benchmark.

Think of your benchmarks. Write them down. What were you interested in? What kind of things did you want to achieve? Were you interested in a particular musical instrument, writing poetry, a particular sport, or a particular activity that you never quite got around to doing?

Perhaps you wanted to learn how to quilt or paint or write but never had time. You wanted to become good at horticulture and learn all about different plants and how to landscape your yard. Or, maybe you were interested in marine life or outer space, but you never had time to study the solar system. Some of you may have been interested in astrology or the study of fossils. How many of you wanted to learn how to play the piano but didn't have the opportunity? Chapter 2 in this book about Happy Things to do in Healthy Aging is a good reference for new ideas.

It is never too late.

The physical dexterity required, as well as the mental practice, will stimulate your mind more than you ever thought possible.

I have many patients who learned how to use the computer at an older age. They took evening courses at senior citizen centers on how to use the computer, just like my 83 year old sister did. They became involved in on-line discussion groups on subjects that interested them, and opened up the entire world to their exploration and fascination. You, too, can become involved in the WEB and discover things you never dreamed off. All you have to do is type any word or phrase about any subject in one or more search engines and you will find more web sites than you can read about on that subject. (Do not divulge any personal information or financial information on blog sites there are a lot of worldwide scam artists waiting to take your money.)

You know, a lot of people travel when they get older. They see as much of the world as they can. How about getting all the information you possibly can about a particular place you are going to visit. If you visit many different places, find out about its ancient history, its culture, and the turbulent times it went through from conquests, to rebuilding, to cultural attitudes, their clothes, the type of food they cooked. You can really get carried away in ancient civilizations. On my transatlantic cruise, many of the people I talked to were in their 70s and some in their 80's. They were sharp and fascinating to talk to. I ended up teaching the ballroom dance classes on the ship because the instructors missed the ship. There were people in their 60's to late 70's learning ballroom dancing and loving it. We switched partners every couple of minutes and everyone was laughing and having a good time.

In my travels through the Maritime Provinces in Canada, I met a lady that was in her mid-sixties. Originally from Northern California, she gave away her belongings, rented her house and decided to see the world. She said "what am I going to do, do the same thing I've been doing over and over?" She decided that the variety of experiences in different regions of the USA and Canada would be very good for her spirit and mental wellbeing, and she was right. She told me that now she has to think constantly about her daily existence, where she is going to go in her van RV, where she would stay, how to navigate different cities, explore what there was to see there etc. Just like the rats in the stimulating environments with new things being put in, her mind was constantly being stimulated by the new places. To keep her company in her RV she bought a small terrier that became a perfect travel companion. She spends her evenings reading or working part time on her graphic design business. When she finds somewhere she likes, she stays there a few weeks to get a feel for the area and participates in local activities.

The world is a very large place. Much larger than that stupid TV screen in front of you. Those nonstop commercials are turning you into a zombie, purchasing anything that has been programmed into your mind. Do you know that it now takes seeing something 14 times in an advertisement before you will act on that product? It used to be just 7 times. That's why there are commercials everywhere, from your smart phone to your gas station pump.

You know, garbage in, garbage out. Just think how much garbage you read in the newspaper or hear on the news every single day. All you hear about is negative events. Is that healthy for your mind? What about the Optimists' creed I read to you, or the positive attitude that is essential for the healthy mind. You are poisoning yourself by filling your mind with negative information that is constantly bombarding you through the news media. Put that aside. Or, if you are going to do it, use it for specific purposes that are mentally and intellectually stimulating.

You can stimulate your mind in thousands of ways, you just have to be creative. There are hundreds of places to find inspiration, from the internet to the reference section of your library. Look in the occupational handbook for all different types of occupations. For a long time, I was interested in sailing, boating, scuba diving, and marine life. I spent a great deal of time learning everything I possibly could about those topics. Once I learned them, I moved onto another subject, about which I knew very little, and tried to educate myself.

When I retired, I went back to college and learned how to program and develop a website. I learned all the ins and outs of a web site's HTML programming and design. It was another area of my mind that was not developed and I forced myself to learn new things.

You should be doing the same thing, constantly adding data to your memory banks, constantly increasing the RAM inside your brain. By increasing the RAM, you will increase your processing speed and you will be able to make connections, and rational thought processes faster. (Jessie, at 94 years old even knew the names of the USA president and the Canadian Prime Minister.)

Throw in a good attitude and a loving heart and you will have a winning combination for the happy mind. By constantly stimulating you mind you are protecting your neurons.

You are keeping them from atrophying. You are also producing something called brain-derived growth factor. You see, this growth factor is just like a growth hormone. It is produced by the brain, and stimulated by mental activity which nurtures your dendrites and helps them grow. It's kind of like having sex.

You need a stimulus for sexual arousal, which is foreplay, the looks, the smell, the ambience, the attractiveness of the other person, etc. You also need a stimulus for brain growth factor arousal, which is a challenging and stimulating mental environment. That stimulus gets the growth factor aroused and says, "Hey, I'm turned on. Let's make some more brain cells. Let's get some more endorphins pumping in here so I feel great." It's a chain reaction, like the "smile awhile and soon the smile gets more smiles." The brain likes it. If the brain is happy, you are happy because you remember things, you feel invigorated, you have lots of energy, and you have lots of stamina. It all starts in the mind. You have to jump start it by stimulating your mind.

Once you have learned something about one subject or discipline, such as math, archeology, playing a musical instrument or learning a language, go to a totally different area of interest and develop that section of your brain. It is like going to the gym, you have to exercise each muscle group; if you do not use those muscles they will deteriorate. Last week I went for a long walk over a large bridge with my daughter. She goes to a fancy gym and takes stretching and core classes. As we were rapidly walking, she was having trouble keeping up with me and started falling behind. She said "Dad, you're in such good shape, I guess I have to start doing cardio exercises." Her cardio endurance deteriorated even though she was limber and had core strength. The same thing happens with the brain, it deteriorates selectively. It loses brain fibers in areas that are not being used, going back to the Use It or Lose It Principle.

If you only use a small portion of your brain to do a few things, the other parts of your brain will wither. What happens if you put your arm in a cast for a few months and don't use it? The muscles atrophy and the arm become weaker. Remember from previous chapters, you have to constantly use those things to keep them healthy. You need to do the same thing with your brain.

The reason I advocate changing topics is because a different topic and a different field of interest will in effect prop up or buttress those areas of your brains that are lacking in stimulation.

Maybe you should go out each week and do a different activity or something different every day of the week. Wouldn't that be interesting? Just like they did with those rats, when they changed their environment every single day or the lady traveling in her motor home. You could also join meetup groups on the internet in different fields of interest.

Man is not designed to live in a retirement complex with nothing but old people sitting around in chairs not talking to each other. Humans are designed to live in environments made up of large varieties of stimuli, and be socially engaged either through family or a network of friends. Old people living with young children, old people living with pets, old people getting out to different environments (not just the mall), old people playing games, traveling, living life to the fullest.

The thing that is wrong with growing old gracefully is that you become the old-old. You want to be the young-old.

For those who just sit around playing Scrabble or Pinochle with their friends, the only part of their brain that will stay developed is the Scrabble or Pinochle part. What about listening to Chopin, Shubert, jazz or seeing that Monet painting in the museum? Have you learned about art history yet, and the different eras that various art forms evolved from? Do you know the different styles of the artists? Traditions of the Samurai, the mediaeval knights? Confucianism? How about the latest ideas on Gestalt therapy, Existentialism, the Envy mind theory, new thoughts on substance abuse, eating disorders, or the local dance company's interpretation of Swan Lake? Or, going to a swing dance with all ages dancing? All those things stimulate different portions of your brain.

You can also read the program manuals and figure out how to get the most out of all the programs you have in your computer and learn to data mine resources on the internet. Talk about mental stimulation, that would certainly get your brain going and allow you to possibly make better investments and lifestyle decisions.

You can do it.

All it takes is the will to do it the will to live life to its fullest, the will to be a young-old instead of an old-old. The baby boomers do not want to get old. They want to stay physically active. They want to stay mentally active. They want to continue to have fun and live life to its fullest. The only way to do it is to continue stimulating and using your mind in all its aspects. Prevent the atrophy that happens with age. Promote a stimulating environment. Live in a stimulating environment.

Live in a place populated with people of all ages, different ideas, different stimuli, and different lifestyles. Do you realize that old farts who do nothing, who live in deed-restricted communities looking for deed violations, who think of no one but themselves, are aging their brains prematurely because they're not open to new ideas? They're not accepting of other lifestyles. They're not even accepting of taller shrubs, slightly dirty roofs or different colors of houses. How dull can you be?

That's the kind of stuff that ages you, ladies and gentlemen, lack of acceptance and lack of diversity. Always the same old/ same old makes you same old, boring, and old. You want to live among artists. You want to live among creativity and life. You want to live in an environment that is stimulating and uplifting with as little stress as possible and as little discord among people as possible.

Live and let live. Enjoy life. Accept diversity among others. Learn from that diversity. Don't complain. Be happy. Look at the positive aspect of everything you see. Look at the beauty in the sky, the birds. Have you ever thought about the flight patterns of birds, and why they migrate? I talked about it a little bit with the pineal gland a few chapters ago and in chapter 2. How about the mating patterns of the bullfrog? Or a clam? If you don't like bullfrogs, then amuse yourself with the unique courtship behavior of the bowerbird.

Some of you may be saying, come on, this is getting a little far-fetched. Well, it isn't. I am trying to get you to stimulate your mind in as many ways as possible to have a longevity mind.

I want you to pay attention to the environment around you. Give your brain a jump-start. Change your routine daily. Expose yourself to a new environment daily. Do different things every day, not the same routine.

On this book rewrite trip I had no set travel plans. I made things up as I went along and visited people and places that gave me further insight into how to improve my old book *Seven Secrets of Anti-Aging* which I renamed *Happy Life Healthy Aging*. In Prince Edward Island, Canada, I met a retired couple from Germany traveling in their RV. They shipped their small motorhome over and in five months traveled over 33,000 kilometers (20,000 miles). They went across Canada all the way to Anchorage Alaska and back. They will ship their RV back to Germany because they like exploring Europe as well. The couple was parked next to me, so I became curious about their German license plate and started talking to them. Through the day the lady was constantly reading something.

Now you're saying, "Okay, okay. I've had enough data. Now tell me what to do."

Here it is.

Read as much as you can about a variety of subjects. Make sure the subjects are diverse, just like the previously mentioned examples. Try something that is mathematical and technical. Then change the next subject to psychological or physiological. Get involved in the arts, which are highly brain stimulating. Be involved in human interactions around young, exciting, different thinking people. Get outside your comfort zone. Explore the universe just like that German couple is doing. They went outside their comfort zone and started exploring places they have never been to before.

Remember I told you to make a list of things you have always been interested in but never had time to pursue. Well, when are you going to make time?

The time is now. Make that list. Make it as long as possible because the longer the list, the longer you will have something to look forward to. If you have something new to look forward to every single day of your life, something that is exciting, your mind is going to be excited. The endorphin levels are going to be high. You are going to be full of life. Your quality of life will increase exponentially.

You've heard of the empty nest syndrome. People downsize and sell their homes because they don't need the room anymore. They buy a small condominium or townhouse. All of a sudden, they have nothing to do. With the kids grown, they've lost their purpose in life. At that stage in life many divorces also occur.

You have to regain that purpose through new experiences. By pursuing new interests, new enthusiasms, and new facts, you will keep your mind healthy and young. That, coupled with physical activity, will stimulate those brain growth factors, protect you from free radical damage, sprout those new neurons to produce new dendrites and increase the connectors in your brain. But you have to do it. No matter what I say, unless you get out there and do it, your mind will not stay young. Did you know that fifty percent of brain cells are already gone when someone is diagnosed with Alzheimer's disease? You want to constantly stimulate that mind to grow new cells in order to have a greater reserve of cells to function with.

Throughout this book, I have talked about the natural approaches towards longevity. Yes, there are different drugs and chemicals that artificially try to stimulate your mind. The problem is, I am not sure what else they may be doing to you. You may be destroying yourself in the long run. Any benefits are short lived so far.

Stick to the natural approaches. Stimulate your mind and get involved emotionally through loving your spouse, your neighbor, your pet. Do good deeds, which will bring further happiness to the environment around you.

What about play time? Play time, I believe, is just as important as mental stimulation for the healthy mind. It stimulates the limbic system, the fun system, the emotional system, the gut feeling you get of pure pleasure when you do something you enjoy.

What you want are positive emotions, like cheerfulness, overall happiness, and the joy of living. A lot of that comes from doing fun things, both individually and in group activities.

Social interaction through volunteering, interest groups, dancing or sport is important because it falls into this limbic, gut-reaction activity level. It falls under this having fun category. It hones your interactive skills. It stimulates you to new thoughts, as well as random thoughts and the inventing of ideas. Bantering back and forth is healthy. It gives you an interest, a pizzazz. Did you ever wonder why people love to gossip? It gives them an emotional high. It gets their juices running. Even gossip is a longevity technique as long as it is not destructive.

We have to do fun things to stimulate our emotions. Figure out what is fun for you. Make that list of things you have always wanted to do or are interested in, re-read chapter two. Have you ever thought of making a list of people you want to associate with or people you wanted to know? I bet you never thought of that, did you?

Make a list of the type of people you want to hang around with; the interests they have, their activity level, their intellectual level, their educational level, their past life experiences, their attitudes towards life. That is as important to you in older age as it is to the teenager making friends.

You know the old saying, the type of people you hang around with, that's the kind of person you are going to become. Think about it, you know you've told your children to stay away from undesirable people or people who are bad influences.

But what about you when you're getting older? Why don't you follow your own advice? Stay away from people who are bad influences on you. Stay away especially from negative people. They'll wear you out and take you down with them.

Chronic complainers are chronic complainers. Who wants to hear that? You want to hang around with people who are young in mind and young in spirit, full of life, ideas, and vitality. People who love to have fun. People who are physically active in all types of sports and people who especially stay mentally active. You may even choose friends who have different levels of activity just so you are exposed to different stimuli. You choose your friends. After all, you have free will. You don't have to be stuck with the same people over and over again.

You're probably asking, "How do you select people as friends? How do you get out of this rut of people doing the same thing with the same people?" You do it by taking charge of your actions.

Go through the list of things you always wanted to do or things you may be possibly interested in. Look for clubs, internet meetup groups and organizations that do those things. Join those clubs or organizations, be it an antique car group, a ring finders metal detection group, a Porsche rally group, a rollerblading group, or the local Writer's Guild. Find out where these organizations are, go to their meetings, meet the people, find the people you like, and start doing things with them. It's a lot easier than you think. Of course, you have to be mobile to do that, so you need to follow the advice in the physical activity section of this book.

It is of utmost importance to maintain physical activity, maintain joint stability, and prevent aches and pains so you can do a variety of things. Everything is a cascade of events. You have to go from point A to get to point B, point B to get to point C. You can't skip things just by taking a magic pill. You've got to put effort into your longevity program to get results.

In the library at Memorial University, in St John's, Newfoundland, I met a doctor writing a thesis. She complained to me that her patients expect her to just give them a pill to fix everything and don't take responsibility for their health. That does not work; the universe does not work that way. You have to do preventive maintenance on everything in this world including your mind and your body.

Your longevity program will be a lot of fun especially if you choose things that you are really interested in. You will have interesting friends, an interesting lifestyle, and all types of things to be involved in. Your time will be so full you will wonder how you ever had time to work before. You will have an action-packed, fun-filled retirement; or should I say, a new vocation, which is a happy life in healthy aging.

Let's just change the topic slightly and talk about staying partially active in your career to prevent aging. You have seen people have midlife crises where they completely quit what they're doing in the middle of their life, in their forties or fifties, and take on a totally different occupation. That happens because people are bored, their work is not stimulating, or they have always had an interest in something else and they feel they are financially capable of pursuing that interest.

Your healthy aging mind program could also involve staying active in your career. If you have a job that is mentally stimulating and interesting, why quit? Stay in your job or career on a part-time basis, but make sure you are doing something you enjoy doing. Life is too short to be miserable working at a job you don't enjoy. It is absolutely pertinent that you get a boost out of what you do for a living. You have to feel you really like doing your job.

I remember going through my practice. Yes, there are ups and downs, there are certain people you don't care to see because they are downers, but, overall, I remember many times going into my practice saying, boy, I really love what I'm doing, this is so much fun.

I especially liked my chelation/nutritional patients because those people were older and so full of life. A lot of the ideas I am telling you about in this book I have learned from observing my successful older patients who came to me to maintain their health and stay young.

I interviewed them extensively. My medical history questionnaire was very thorough. It covered everything: How many kids they've had, how many spouses they've had, whether or not they're happy, if they've had psychiatric treatment, any ailments, what they did in their careers and their lives. By having such an extensive survey on older people, I was able to observe what worked and what didn't work.

Successful longevity doesn't happen spontaneously. People who are successful in an older age planned their success all along by following anti-aging principles. Through following my patients, the randomness of insights became less random and more consistent. A little research here, a little research there. Comments here and there. An attitude here and an attitude there. From that, you can get a picture of how people do best as they age. You get a picture of how people stay physically active and disease-free as they age. You get a picture of how people stay mentally clear and involved in life as they age. You get a blueprint for a darn good longevity program that is do-able.

What I am telling you is a compilation of current research and observation; things you can do. Yes, you have genes that can affect your outcome to a certain extent. But even if you do have genes stacked against you, you can modify the genetic activity through what you do. The new science of "epigenetics" studies reveal how behavior modifies genes. Just as I have seen in physical activity studies based upon identical twins, I know the same thing is true in all other aspects of healthy aging.

I know people can will themselves to live longer, will themselves to be happy, and will themselves to modify disease processes.

The mind is powerful.

It can be stimulated to produce the right chemicals, produce a happy environment to the cells, and produce growth and the sprouting of new cells. Give the brain adequate oxygenation through increased circulation and physical activity, give it a variety of mental stimulation and it's going to be happy. It's going to be very happy and reward you with a long, prosperous, happy life. If you like what you are doing in your job, why quit? Stay working on a part time basis. It's great for your pocketbook too, because then you don't have to dip into your retirement savings all the time. If you have plenty of money, give the extra money away to charity or provide a scholarship for a needy child who is mentally gifted and cannot afford the tuition for the university.

There is a lot of good you can do in society. By volunteering your expertise or your professional time you are helping society as a whole and giving back.

You can make time to do anything you want to do, especially after you retire. Get a part-time job, something you love to do in your new area that you move to; or, do volunteer work for a worthy cause, or just spend your time doing a variety of activities you enjoy. The "Happy Things to do in Healthy Aging" chapter should give you some ideas of things to try.

I figured, for me, it was better to work on a part-time basis in my profession for a while and then retire after a few years when newer interests developed. Since I love medicine, I stay active in my specialty of physical medicine and rehabilitation through volunteering at a free clinic. I also go to weekly continuing medical education seminars in my area to stay current in medicine.

In retirement, after a while, you get tired of playing golf or deep sea fishing; then, you say to yourself, "What else is there to do?" If you pace yourself in a progressive longevity program, make your list of things that you want to do, keep yourself mentally active, learn new things and stay physically active, your mind and your body should stay young.

In 2005 a study was published in the *New England Journal of Medicine* on the risk of dementia and leisure time activity. They found that reading, playing board games, playing a musical instrument and dancing were associated with a lower risk of dementia. Frequency made a difference; the more you did those things, the better the outcome. Dancing was the only physical activity in that study associated with a lower risk of dementia. In evaluating the data, dancing had the lowest risk. The study backs up everything that I wrote in my *Dance to Live* book. So, if you get tired of playing golf why not try dancing? It increases neuroplasticity (the ability to make quick, instantaneous decisions by the brain, creating new neural pathways as needed), and it keeps you physically fit.

Even if you have a disease where you cannot be as mobile as you want, push yourself, do rehabilitative exercise. We plan to have a whole series of neck, back, knee, foot, hand, shoulder etc. joint rehabilitation exercises available on our website *www.happylifehealthyaging.com* Use them, after asking your doctor. Resurface your joints. Strengthen your muscles and bones. Get back on track. But, keep your mind going. Keep it interested. Keep it diverse. Learn new things. Continue doing the fun things you used to love to do. Associate with fun-loving, interesting people and you will have a blast into your silver years.

If you are in a stressful environment, get out of it. Life is too short to put up with a stressful environment. You have decision-making abilities. It is your life you are playing with. Do something about it.

Surround yourself with stress-free people, stress-free environments, and a fun-filled mentally stimulating environment. Do a variety of things. Change your activity every day. Have new stimuli every day. Make a list for 365 days of the year what you are going to do and go through that list and follow through. If that's too long, make a thirty-day list, or even a seven-day list. Just do it.

Set new goals for yourself. Write down what you want to do every month, every year, and pursue those goals. The important thing is that you write those goals down, write those lists down, and check them off as you do them. Be methodical. This way, you will stimulate every single part of your brain. You know, this whole program is free. Libraries don't cost much. All you need is a pair of walking shoes and a desire to stay young. What you put into your mind is just as important as what you put into your mouth. Garbage in is garbage out.

If you are under a tremendous amount of stress or negative emotions, your body is going to react to it. You will have decreased resistance. You're going to get more illnesses.

There were studies done in Britain where people were exposed to a cold virus. The ones under the highest stress had the highest incidents of catching a cold. Stress reduces the power of your immune system to protect itself and you are much more susceptible to any disease process that comes along. As I mentioned in the introduction, stress has been linked to just about every disease of our modern society, from cancer to heart disease to high blood pressure, stroke, skin conditions, allergies, you name it, it can be stress induced.

Dr. Hans Selye did an excellent job in his book, *The Stress of Life* in pointing out how prolonged stress can gradually destroy our immune system. It has to do with the cortisol level, which, when unchecked, gradually reduces our immunity and slowly kills us.

You need to counteract stressful situations by getting out of them. Eliminate anything in your life that prevents you from having happy thoughts and peace of mind. You are in charge. You are not a victim of circumstance. You can always change the circumstances around you. Sometimes a small change can make a big difference to your peace of mind. You are in charge.

You can even change your inner thought processes by visualizing happier times in your life, which will put you in a relaxed state and help boost your immune system.
Get funny movies and watch them to reduce your stress level. Laughter therapy has been shown to be successful in beating even the greatest

diseases. Of course, one of the best ways to reduce stress is to engage in play time doing things that you love to do, be it dancing, bicycling, bird watching, or any activity that gives you great physical pleasure. My friend, the executive of a corporation with his own private jet, removed himself from the stress. He just quit. All his friends are six-feet under. But he was able to break free of the stressful situation, quit his job and live a happy, stress-free existence sailing in Florida.

He changed his destiny, and so can you. Put some time and thought into it. What can you do to change your environment, reduce your stress load, and stimulate your mind? I have always thought the work week was a little screwed up. We work five days a week and have two days off.

How about if we turn it around? Work two days a week and have five days off. Wouldn't that be a wonderful situation to be in, work part-time and play most of the time? (See chapter 2) The play time would certainly reduce your stress level allowing you to pursue all kinds of interests, stimulating different areas of the brain that needed a tune-up to stay young. The job environment can also be a volunteer position in which you use your past skills to teach others to become successful in those skills. When we feel needed and appreciated, we will get a lot more out of the job environment and we will contribute a lot more toward that job environment.

Remember, happy thoughts are essential toward a successful longevity program. Mental stimulation is essential in healthy aging. Stress reduction is essential for healthy longevity as well as physical activity.

Stress to your body is like toxins in your food. Toxins poison you slowly. Stress poisons your mind and destroys your body slowly also.

Happy thoughts, mental stimulation, and peace of mind are the magic pills that keep you healthy. The healthy aging mind is a happy mind. It is a stress-free mind. It is a stimulated mind. It is an inquisitive mind. It is a mind that loves to have social interaction, a mind that wants to continually learn new things, a mind that is continually developing, a mind that is happy. Whatever the mind can conceive, it can achieve. If you truly want a longevity program that keeps you young well into your nineties and over a hundred, the time to start action is now. You can do it. Only you can do it.

The other alternatives are not very pleasing. You do not want to reserve that bed in the nursing home when you're seventy. You don't want to reserve that bed at all. You want to stay active until you drop dead at 105.

You are living through a revolution, a revolution of changes in thoughts and attitudes. A revolution in what aging means to us. You want to stay young forever. You want to stay physically active, be mentally worthwhile, and have a phenomenal quality of life. You can do it. You can do it.

Do it now. Right now.

CONCLUSION

Let's go over what we have covered in this book and try to meld it altogether for you; kind of like a cheeseburger where the cheese has melted into the meat. Or, for you vegetarians, natural fruit and yogurt combined in a blender.

As you think about the key features of this book, you will realize that Happy Life Healthy Aging requires some effort. Healthy longevity requires some planning. It can be a whole bunch of fun because the rewards are tangible. You can feel the rewards. You can feel yourself staying younger, becoming younger, losing weight, having more energy and being mentally sharp. You can feel yourself developing a zest for life, a quest for knowledge, greater muscle strength, greater physical endurance, and an overall peace of mind and happiness with love and passion for what you are doing.

A Maître d' on a cruise ship once told me "There are four things important in life, 1. A love of God 2. Your health 3. Your family and the friends you have 4. A means to make a living." The points he stated are important in that Happy Life in Healthy Aging.

If you follow the longevity program, you will be a better spouse and a better friend to your friends. (Social interaction is very important in longevity.) You will not be a burden on your children. You will lead an active life exploring the wonders of the world, being an asset to society and helping other people. Time will just fly because you are having so much fun.

A patient once told me, "I had no idea I'd be having so much fun and enjoying life as much as I am now that I am retired." How many of you can say that? If you follow this program, you will be saying that. You will say, "Dr. Lenhart, this is fantastic. I never knew I could have so much energy and zest for life. I feel younger now than I did when I was forty."

You have to be willing to change your environment, reduce stress, constantly challenge your mind, hang around positive people and have lots and lots of fun.

When you put everything in this book together, what do you have? The secrets to a happy life in healthy aging.

I want all of you to be like my healthy elderly patients, active, fun-loving, alert, having the best time in their lives ever.

Thank You for reading this book, you may want to read it over again because there is so much information here.

Best Wishes and have a happy life.

Dr. John P. Lenhart

Tell a friend about this book…. It may help them to live a healthier life.

References – Please visit our web site *www.happylifehealthyaging.com* and go to the Reference Section.

ORDERING INFORMATION

This book is available on our web site *www.happylifehealthyaging.com*, amazon.com and other retailers.

For boutique foods, probiotics and supplements, go to the above web site and click on the description and explanation of the product. Products from various high quality manufacturers will be available for comparison. Also visit your local health food store. As scientific research progresses, various companies that we feel have a unique product will be featured.

Don't forget to write to us with all your stories of success, so we can share them with others on our web site. Tell us of the little things you did that made a major impact in your life for keeping you young, the activities you are doing, the fun you are having, and the good deeds you've engaged in. I want every one of you to be happy, healthy, wealthy, wise, prosperous, successful, and in love.

Our E-mail is: *info@happylifehealthyaging.com*

Or: www.happylifehealthyaging@gmail.com

Medfo Publishing

St. Petersburg, Florida USA

—

www.ingramcontent.com/pod-product-compliance
Lightning Source LLC
Chambersburg PA
CBHW062210270326
41930CB00009B/1702

9 781930 822337